Super
Nutrients
H A N D B O O K

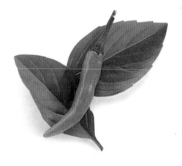

D1444680

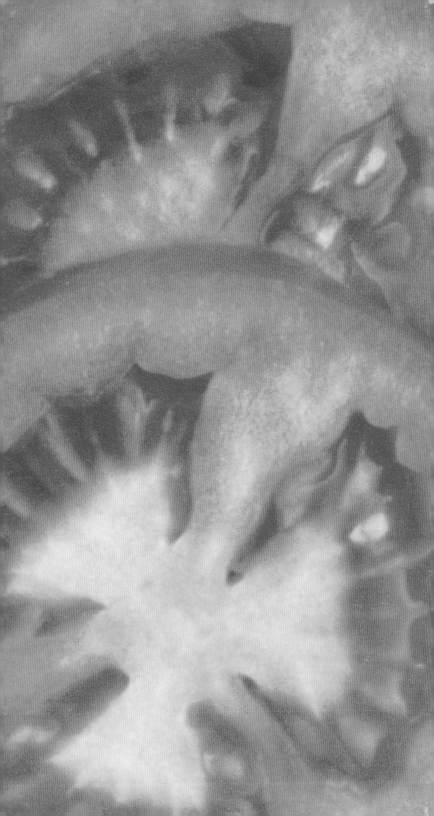

Super
Nutrients
HANDBOOK

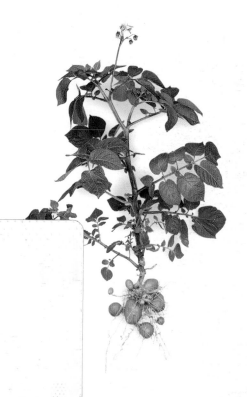

LYNDEL COSTAIN

A Dorling Kindersley Book

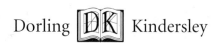

Dorling **DK** Kindersley

LONDON, NEW YORK, SYDNEY, DELHI, PARIS,
MUNICH AND JOHANNESBURG

Project Editor Susannah Steel
Art Editor Alison Lotinga
Managing Editor Gillian Roberts
Managing Art Editor Tracey Ward
Category Publisher Mary-Clare Jerram
Art Director Tracy Killick
DTP Designers Louise Paddick and Louise Waller
Production Manager Maryann Webster
US Editors Barbara Minton and Crystal A. Coble
US Editorial Director LaVonne Carlson

First American Edition 2001
2 4 6 8 10 9 7 5 3 1
Published in the United States by Dorling Kindersley Publishing, Inc.,
95 Madison Avenue, New York, NY 10016

Library of Congress Cataloging-in-Publication Data

Costain, Lyndel.
  Supernutrients handbook : the hidden power in plant foods
that benefit body and mind / Lyndel Costain.
    p. cm.
  Includes index.
  ISBN 0-7894-7179-5 (alk. paper)
    1. Nutrition. 2. Functional foods. 3. Phytochemicals. I. Title.

RA784 .C6224 2001
613.2'62--dc21   00-053107

Color reproduced by Colourscan, Singapore
Printed and bound in Italy by Graphicom

see our complete
catalog at
www.dk.com

Contents

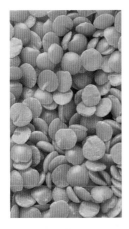
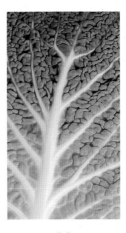
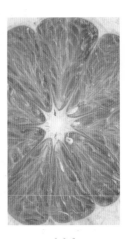

AUTHOR'S
INTRODUCTION

If you are reading this, you probably have a keen interest in food and how it can benefit your health. By the time you've digested what this book has to offer, I hope you will feel positively enthusiastic about the unique power of plant foods.

Why is there so much fuss about fruit and vegetables? One reason is that research keeps unearthing links between a diet rich in plant foods and reduced risk of chronic disease. For example, reviews of more than 150 population studies revealed that people who ate five portions of fruit and vegetables daily were half as likely to develop most types of cancer than people who ate less than two portions a day. Studies also link a regular intake of wholegrains and nuts with a significantly lower risk of heart disease.

FREE-RADICAL FIGHTERS

Plant foods are excellent sources of antioxidants – super nutrients that help to protect the body from potentially damaging free radicals. Some free radicals are important for good health, but excessive or unchecked amounts are implicated in a number of chronic diseases and conditions, including heart disease, cancer, cataracts, Parkinson's and Alzheimer's disease, diabetes, lung disease, arthritis, and multiple sclerosis. There is usually a genetic basis to chronic disease, meaning that some people are more vulnerable to certain diseases or even early aging. A protective diet and environment may help reduce this risk of chronic disease by slowing degenerative processes, which also leads to healthier aging.

WHAT GIVES
PLANTS THEIR POWER?

Plants are a rich source of conventional nutrients such as vitamins, minerals, and carbohydrates. They also contain a vast range of bioactive compounds – organic chemicals that are called phytochemicals ("phyto," meaning plant).

Until the late '80s, phytochemicals mainly interested plant scientists. However, as research began to uncover links between high fruit and vegetable intakes and lower rates of chronic disease, it also revealed that their protective effects could not be explained by conventional nutrients alone. Nutrition scientists are now fascinated by phytochemicals and are working to decide how we can benefit most from what they offer. Many can function as antioxidants; others work in different ways.

Studying phytochemicals is not easy. There is still much to know about familiar ones, and thousands are yet to be investigated that may have even more beneficial effects than those studied to date! Pure forms of single phytochemicals that show a certain activity in a laboratory test tube may work very differently in the body. Phytochemicals also seem to work best in conjunction with nutrients and other phytochemicals.

RESEARCH FINDINGS

This book outlines what scientific research tells us to date about how phytochemicals may function in test tubes, in living cells, and in humans. Since this information has had to be condensed, and at times simplified, it may sometimes make research findings appear more definitive than they really are. For example, if a phytochemical is said to have an "anti-cancer" effect, this does not mean it will prevent or stop cancer, but that phytochemical actions which inhibit the growth of cancer cells in some way have been identified in laboratory settings.

There is also still only very limited evidence about how phytochemicals might directly reduce the incidence of any form of chronic disease. More human intervention studies and techniques to assess phytochemical actions in the body are needed to help scientists draw clearer conclusions about why plant foods are protective (see p.29).

Each phytochemical in this book has its own profile, highlighted by key food sources. After all, the best way to make the most of phytochemicals is to eat whole foods, and it is this overall package that offers the greatest health benefits. Read the introductory pages to each category of phytochemicals, too. This will help you understand the different sections more fully.

OPTIMUM BENEFITS

Because of the complex interactions between nutrients, phytochemicals, and the body itself, it isn't yet possible to state how much of an individual phytochemical is needed for optimal health. In fact, different people may benefit from different amounts, and more research is needed to determine the phytochemical content of foods, which, like vitamins and minerals, can vary according to growing conditions, ripeness, and cooking methods.

I explain all this to help make sure you view the information in the right context. We are dealing with a very new, ever-evolving, and intensely exciting area of nutrition research. The potential for health benefits from phytochemicals, both as part of a healthy diet and as thoroughly researched therapeutic supplements for people with identified health risks, is enormous. And while nutrition scientists are busy gathering and refining this knowledge, we can benefit from the evidence that a diet rich in a variety of fruit, vegetables, and other plant foods is linked to reduced risk of many conditions. It is also a delicious way to safeguard our health and help us all get the best from life.

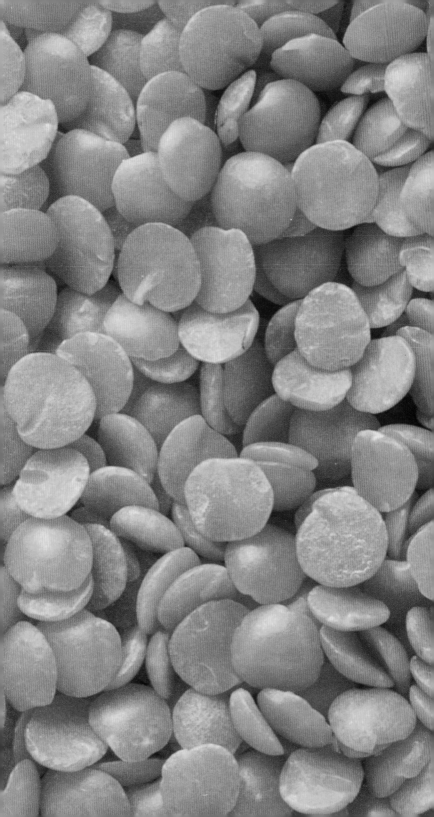

Part One

In an age when we want to look good, live

longer, and feel healthier, compelling research

has revealed the protective power of plant foods

that benefit body and mind. This power comes

from a vast range of nutrients, fiber, and

"phytochemicals."

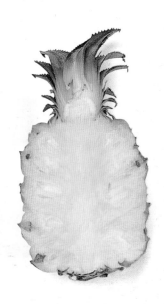

PHYTOCHEMICALS EXPLAINED

Phytochemicals ("phyto" means plant) are biologically active compounds in plants. To date, scientists have identified over 12,000 phytochemicals, and one plant can contain literally hundreds of different types of these compounds.

Phytochemicals define a plant's color and flavor; they are also vital for its health and survival. This is because phytochemicals help plant growth by deterring harmful predators, bacteria, and viruses, protecting against damaging sun rays, and attracting birds and insects to the plant's pretty petals and foliage, which in turn promotes pollination and seed dispersal.

PROTECTING OUR GENERAL HEALTH

The phytochemicals in plants take on a new life when we eat them, working to benefit our health and longevity. In fact, dietitians and nutritionists are clear that eating a balanced diet rich in plant foods will help to reduce the risk of a variety of long-term diseases such as heart disease, stroke, cancer, and cataracts. However, some phytochemicals can be poisonous or taste truly awful – they are present in plants in order to deter animals who might otherwise eat them. With a few exceptions, these "unpleasant" phytochemicals are only found in wild plants and are not part of our

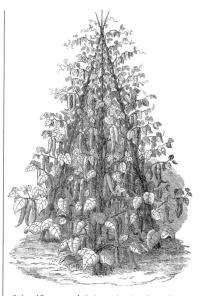

Scientific research is investigating how the phytochemicals in plant foods such as green beans are absorbed and used by the body, and their subsequent effects on human health.

normal diet – although care still needs to be taken with some foods (*see pp.108–113*).

High doses of a number of phytochemicals have pharmacological effects in the body, and even today plants remain important sources of a range of therapeutic drugs. Phytochemicals are the active "ingredients" in herbal medicines, too.

HOW DIFFERENT ARE PHYTOCHEMICALS?

Vitamins, minerals, protein, fat, carbohydrate, and fiber are all essential nutrients, meaning that we must get them from food in order for our bodies to function properly. For example, if we lack vitamin C in our diet we develop a deficiency disease called scurvy which could ultimately lead to death.

Phytochemicals are different from these more familiar food components and are described not as "nutrients," but as "non-nutrient" compounds, since there is currently no evidence to show they are essential to life. For this reason there is no clearly defined recommended intake for different phytochemicals in the way that vitamins, minerals, and other nutrients have Recommended Daily Allowances (RDAs). However, this could all change as research into phytochemicals progresses.

RESEARCHING PLANT FOODS

For decades, plant scientists have been researching phytochemicals in relation to the health benefits plants can give. In 1981 the first report linking diet and cancer was published by two British professors, Sir Richard Doll and Richard Peto, with the suggestion that about 35 percent of all cancers could be caused by diet. This stimulated interest in the role of plant foods in human health, but it is only in the last ten years that phytochemical research has taken off. Compare this to over a century of research into nutrients – though there is still much to learn here, too!

Important publications then triggered a growing fascination with phytochemicals. Between 1982 and 1992 a number of epidemiological reviews (studies that identify, and seek to explain, the incidence of health and disease in a population; *see also p.29*) across Europe and in the U.S. concluded that diet could influence many cancers, and that high fruit and vegetable intakes were linked to a decreased risk.

Then in 1993 came a report from the Zutphen Elderly Study, a study of the health and dietary habits of 800 elderly Dutchmen. After five years, those with the highest intakes of fruit and vegetables containing phytochemicals called flavonoids *(pp.34–35)* had a significantly lower risk of dying from coronary heart disease compared to those with low intakes. This was true even after accounting for other factors that can affect health, namely age, weight, cigarette smoking, blood pressure, blood cholesterol, activity level, and intakes of vitamins C and E, betacarotene, and fiber.

Phytochemical research is now flourishing. Until recently, much research centered on the effects of pure phytochemicals in a laboratory environment; now the focus is on how phytochemicals react in the body, and the search is on for new, beneficial phytochemicals. This will add weight to the existing findings of population and laboratory studies. It will also provide clearer information about optimal food intakes and in what forms and combinations so we can make the most of plant power.

CHANGING DIETARY PATTERNS

Diets in developed countries have changed dramatically over the course of time. Some of the most rapid change has been in the last 50 years, resulting in a wide range of refined foods and lower intakes of plant foods.

The change in the human diet has resulted in a shift from what was an unrefined, low fat, plant food-rich diet that required much hard work to procure, to a highly refined diet that is instantly accessible and often lacking in fruit and vegetables.

ANCESTRAL DIETS

For tens of thousands of years the diet of our hunter-gatherer ancestors was made up of varying proportions of plant foods – root vegetables, leaves, seeds, fruits – and animal foods. Although the food supply

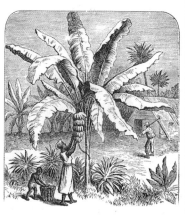

The diet of most people today is generally less healthy than it used to be; we eat fewer wholegrains, vegetables, and fruit than our ancestors did.

wasn't always reliable, their diet would have been rich in nutrients such as folate, vitamin C, omega 3 fats – and phytochemicals. In evolutionary terms we should still, today, be genetically adapted to a diet brimming with diverse plant foods and phytochemicals; the type of diet that seems to allow our body to function at its best. Yet the start of food cultivation and processing marked the beginning of a decline in the variety and quantity of plant foods in human diets.

CULTIVATED CROPS

Farming arrived about 10,000 years ago with the cultivation of crops and a more reliable food supply; wheat, maize, and rice became staple crops in different parts of the world. During the late nineteenth century food processing, preservation, and transportation developed, together with improvements in breeding techniques for plant foods and live-stock. Unleashed, these agricultural and technological advances surged full steam ahead. Since the 1950s, home freezers, microwave ovens, convenience food, one-stop supermarkets, restaurants, and home delivery services have all made their mark. On one hand, we have never had such a variety of foods; on the other, the Western diet is more refined than ever before. We are also far less active.

These diet-related problems are not new to developed countries, but as technology and convenience food enters developing countries and local people move away from their traditional diets, problems will inevitably follow.

NUTRITIONAL RESEARCH

Nutritional research in the 1930s and '40s focused on vitamins, minerals, and general nutrient requirements. This formed the basis for the "four food groups," dietary balance was promoted, and worldwide health problems caused by nutrient deficiencies were addressed.

In the late 1950s, Dr. Ancel Keys began a major study – the Seven Countries Study – to investigate the diet and pattern of disease in 12,000 middle-aged men in Greece, Italy, former Yugoslavia, the Netherlands, Finland, the U.S., and Japan. The findings showed that what we eat can affect our long-term health and highlighted the health benefits of the Mediterranean and Japanese diets *(pp.14-15)*. A whole new interest in diet and health was born and dietary trends took hold: vegetarianism in the 1960s; intensive farming and convenience food in the '70s; "eat less fat and more fiber" in the '80s; optimal health and "wellness" as a focus in the '90s. Meanwhile, chronic

health conditions – such as diabetes, obesity, cancer, osteoporosis, arthritis, and postmenopausal symptoms – have all been on the increase.

Thanks largely to modern medicine, sanitation, and enough food to eat, we live longer than ever before. But our quality of life now is

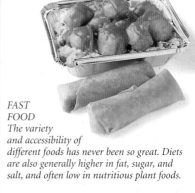

FAST FOOD The variety and accessibility of different foods has never been so great. Diets are also generally higher in fat, sugar, and salt, and often low in nutritious plant foods.

too often affected by poor health. It could be that our changing diet and lifestyle has reached a point where life expectancy has begun to falter.

Plant power, as part of a balanced diet, can help us delay the onset and the severity of such chronic and degenerative conditions and diseases. In fact, research from the U.S. recently highlighted that women who eat in line with dietary recommendations *(p.18)* have a 30 percent lower risk of dying from any cause than women who don't. And the World Cancer Research Fund advises that a diet rich in a variety of fruit and vegetables could prevent at least 20 percent of all cancers. Fortunately, nutritional research, public nutrition education, and people's increasing knowledge about how to eat well is steering us in the right direction.

TRADITIONAL DIETARY PATTERNS

Plants have been viewed as healing foods for thousands of years. Garlic was a favorite of the Greeks, Romans, and Egyptians; ginger was used extensively throughout Asia; and olive oil was revered by the Minoan civilizations of Crete.

The health benefits of three classic cuisines – the Mediterranean diet, the Japanese diet, and the vegetarian diet – are supported by a large body of population and clinical studies. With the global variety of foods now available to us, it is has never been easier to maximize these benefits.

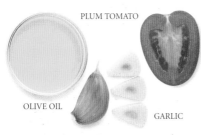

PLUM TOMATO

OLIVE OIL

GARLIC

FLAVORFUL INGREDIENTS
Oil, garlic, and tomatoes are vital ingredients of the Mediterranean diet, along with an abundance of vegetables, legumes, herbs, wholegrains, nuts, fruit, and fish.

THE MEDITERRANEAN DIET

The Mediterranean diet hails from the dietary traditions of populations bordering the Mediterranean sea. Olive oil is the main source of fat, and wine is the favorite beverage. It is a vibrantly colorful cuisine and full of satisfying flavor, with only small amounts of poultry, meat, and dairy products. It is associated with

a lower risk of coronary heart disease, high blood pressure, diabetes, and certain cancers. A study showed that when adopted by Westerners recovering from a heart attack, a Mediterranean-style diet was more heart protective than a low fat diet.

The traditional Mediterranean diet is low in cholesterol-raising saturated fat and rich in powerful plant foods. In fact, the recommendation by the World Health Organization to eat at least five portions of fruit and vegetables daily was based on the Mediterranean diet and its association with a low risk of chronic diseases.

THE JAPANESE DIET

Compared to the West, the long-lived Japanese enjoy lower rates of coronary heart disease, obesity, breast and prostate cancer, osteoporosis-induced hip fracture, and menopausal symptoms. Japanese people living in Western countries have similar health problems to their local compatriots, suggesting that diet and lifestyle play a major role in the Japanese health advantage. Sadly, incoming Western food habits are now influencing health in Japan.

The traditional Japanese diet centers on rice, soy beans, fish, seafood, and vegetables. Noodles, seaweed, spices, and fruit are also enjoyed, and meat is used more as a garnish or to flavor sauces. Presentation is paramount. Its only drawback is its high salt content. Fish and soy beans provide a good supply of essential omega 3 fats (*p.22*). And the humble soy bean (*p.50*), the focus of recent nutritional research, no doubt contributes to the benefits of the Japanese and other Asian diets.

THE VEGETARIAN DIET

About five percent of Western populations now claim to be vegetarian. Studies on the diet and health of

VEGETARIAN STIR FRY
A number of cultures and religions follow vegetarian diets, and vegetarianism is also popular for moral, ethical, and health reasons.

vegetarians in Britain and the U.S. confirm that vegetarian diets tend to be lower in saturated fat (but not necessarily total fat), and richer in fiber and phytochemicals than the diets of omnivores. Vegetarians also tend to be slimmer, suffer less from high blood pressure, diabetes, and gallstones, and have lower rates of heart disease. You don't need to be strictly vegetarian to enjoy similar health benefits; the fact that a variety of plant foods forms the bulk of this diet (a vegan diet contains only plant foods), rather than simply not eating meat, seems to be the key.

JAPANESE INGREDIENTS
The traditional Japanese diet of low fat, plant-based foods is so healthy that nutritionists in Japan are trying to dissuade the population from adopting a Western diet (also an issue in Mediterranean countries).

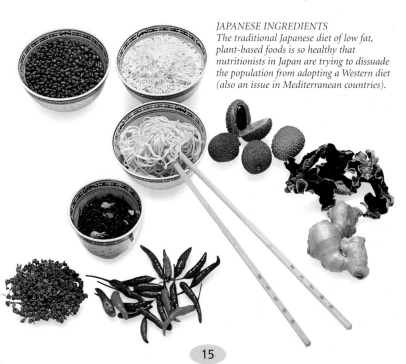

KEY FUNCTIONS OF PHYTOCHEMICALS

Our parents were quite right when they told us to eat our greens. Research into phytochemicals in fruit, vegetables, and other plant foods is already revealing a range of mechanisms to explain how they might work to protect our health.

It is clear that plant foods are good for our health – and the phytochemicals they contain are partly responsible. What is less clear is exactly why this is. In laboratory studies, and some human studies *(p.29)*, different phytochemicals have been shown to have the following types of effects *(see also glossary and entries in Part Two for more details)*:

• Antioxidant
• Anticancer
• Anti-inflammatory
• Antithrombotic
• Antibacterial, antiviral, antifungal
• Cholesterol lowering
• Hormone influencing
• Blood vessel relaxing
• Immune system stimulating
• Gut bacteria balancing.

ANTIOXIDANTS EXPLAINED

A number of these phytochemical effects may be due to their influence on enzymes, others are linked to their ability to work as antioxidants. An antioxidant protects against the effects of oxidation. Think of it in terms of a rusty iron nail. Oxygen in the air reacts with iron to form rust. Oxygen can also react with fat, say in butter, and turn it rancid. As we all breathe in oxygen, similar oxygen-related processes happen in our body. And without the protective effects of antioxidants, these unchecked oxygen reactions could "rust" our bodies over time.

FREE RADICALS

Every cell in the body uses oxygen to produce energy and allow the body to function *(p.20)*. This is a normal part of the body's metabolism. While all these oxygen reactions are happening, very unstable molecules known as "free radicals" can be produced. Free radicals are unstable because they are missing an electron. However, they are very quick to snatch an electron from somewhere else in the body – for example, from a body cell – to help them become stable again. This action can damage body cells and also trigger the formation of another free radical, and so a chain reaction starts.

Antioxidants can save the day by giving up one of their own electrons and neutralizing free radicals. This stops cell damage and eventually the chain reaction.

Free radicals are also deliberately made by the cells of our immune system to help destroy invading bacteria and viruses. Free radicals are also increased in the body by pollution, UV sunlight, radiation, cigarette smoke, stress, and excess polyunsaturated fat. Overall, we are exposed to around ten million free radical "hits" every day. The body produces some antioxidants, but damage can develop if free radical production becomes excessive. This is called "oxidative stress." Damage caused by oxidative stress accumulates with age, and some scientists believe that early aging and chronic health problems (e.g., cancer, heart disease, cataracts, rheumatoid arthritis, Alzheimer's disease) are initiated by free radical damage, then take years to develop. The body's ability to produce its own antioxidants may also decline with age. Finally, different antioxidants may neutralize free radicals in different parts of the body and regenerate one another. This means that getting a range of different antioxidants from a variety of foods throughout our lifetime is very important.

The antioxidant defense system limits free radicals from:
• Damaging cholesterol-carrying particles, known as low-density lipoprotein or "bad" LDL cholesterol, which may increase the risk of atherosclerosis.
• Contributing to the formation of blood clots (thrombosis), which may increase the risk of a heart attack or stroke) over time.
• Damaging a cell's genetic material (DNA), which may lead to cancer.
• Triggering inflammation.
• Suppressing the immune system.
• Impairing cell function.
Defending against all these effects may slow the progression of chronic disease and aging.

CANCER-FIGHTING PHYTOCHEMICALS

One in three people will develop cancer at some time in their lives. Cancers can start when the DNA or genetic material in cells is damaged (known as "initiation") by carcinogens. Years may pass before the cancer becomes noticeable. Cancerous cells grow in an unrestrained way, invade and damage healthy tissues, and can spread to other parts of the body, forming secondary growths (metastases). Some phytochemicals seem to stimulate enzymes that block carcinogens or suppress this spread of cancer cells. Others with antioxidant effects may help the immune system to remain strong and destroy any damaged cells.

CHOOSING A BALANCED DIET

Food is our fuel; it also protects, nourishes, and gives great pleasure. Getting our fuel mix right is vital for good health. Fruit and vegetables provide a unique phytochemical edge, but they aren't enough for a complete balanced diet.

We need to eat a wide variety of different foods each day to make sure we have all the nutrients our bodies need and to keep our taste buds satisfied! In order to provide a healthy variety in your diet, make that you choose foods from each of the five food segments as outlined in the wheel of food *(see right)*. This way of eating is suitable for older children and adults *(for young children, see p.116)*.

HOW MUCH TO EAT – dependant on age, sex, and activity levels

	MAIN NUTRIENTS	WHAT TO CHOOSE
BREAD, POTATOES, & OTHER CEREALS	Carbohydrate (mainly starchy), fiber, B vitamins, potassium, selenium, some protein, iron, and calcium, phytochemicals, and vitamin E.	All kinds of bread, pasta, rice, noodles, breakfast cereals, potatoes, yams, oats, and grains. Aim for three daily servings of wholegrain types.
FRUIT & VEGETABLES	Vitamin C, folate, betacarotene, fiber, magnesium, potassium, some carbohydrate, iron, and calcium, phytochemicals.	All types – fresh, frozen, canned, dried, and juices. Choose from a variety of different types and colors every day.
MILK & DAIRY FOODS & ALTERNATIVES	Calcium, protein, vitamins A, B2, B12, and D, zinc, phytochemicals in soy-based foods.	Opt for low-fat varieties, e.g., reduced fat milk, yogurt, fromage frais, cheeses, and calcium-fortified soy milk or yogurt.
MEAT, FISH & ALTERNATIVES	Protein, iron, B vitamins, zinc, magnesium, potassium, phytochemicals in peas, beans, lentils, nuts, seeds, and tofu.	Lean and trimmed meats, poultry, all types of fish, eggs, beans, split peas and lentils, nuts, and meat substitutes, e.g., tofu.
FOODS RICH IN FAT AND/OR SUGAR	Sugars and fats, including some essential fats, vitamins, and minerals, phytochemicals in oils, e.g., virgin olive oil, sesame oil, wholewheat crackers, and chocolate.	Unsaturated oils, e.g., olive, rapeseed, sunflower, soy and their spreads. Use fats sparingly when preparing food.

Each segment represents one of the five main food groups that constitute a balanced diet. Foods in each group are good sources of similar nutrients and so can be interchanged. The size of the segments varies according to the healthiest proportions for each food group in your diet. Note that plant foods – fruit, vegetables, breads, potatoes, and cereals – make up two thirds of the wheel. By following these general guidelines you will automatically be choosing a diet that is high in energy-giving carbohydrate, moderate in protein and fat (but low in saturated fat), and rich in vitamins, minerals, and phytochemicals.

Health experts world-wide now promote this balance and variety of foods as the ideal way to eat to keep in shape, stay fit, and reduce your risk of ill health; in other words, to help you get the best from life.

WHEEL OF FOOD

HOW MUCH	OTHER POINTS
Make these the basis of each meal, but limit added fat. One serving is: 1 slice of bread; ½ bagel; bowl of cereal; ⅓ cup cooked rice, ½ cup pasta or noodles. Have at least 6 servings each day.	Most people would benefit from eating more of these foods. They are filling, nutritious, and not fattening as is commonly believed. Fruit buns, biscuits, cereal, and crackers make good snacks.
Aim for 5-9 portions every day. One portion is: 2 tbsp. vegetables, 2-3 tbsp. cooked fruit, side salad, medium fruit, 1 glass of juice, 1 tbsp. dried fruit.	Most people could benefit from eating more. Diets rich in fruit and vegetables can help protect against chronic disease and aid weight control.
Eat or drink a moderate amount, e.g., 2-3 servings daily. One serving is 6oz. milk/soy milk, 1 small pot yogurt, 1oz. cheese, or 4oz. cottage cheese.	A good calcium intake throughout life (especially during adolescence and in the early twenties) helps reduce risk of osteoporosis.
Eat moderate amounts, e.g., 2–3 servings per day. One serving is: 2–3oz. meat, 4oz. fish, 1–2 eggs, 3–4 tbsp. cooked beans/lentils, or 2oz. nuts.	Important in helping to prevent iron deficiency that is most common among women of child-bearing age and under fives.
Eat foods high in fat and/or sugar in small amounts, especially those high in saturated fat. Look for lower fat alternatives to spreads, dressings, and ready-made meals.	Keep any sugary foods and drinks to mealtimes to reduce the risk of tooth decay. Diets high in saturated fat are linked to an increased risk of heart disease.

WHAT IS IN PLANT FOODS?

Food is made up of carbohydrate, fats, protein, fiber, vitamins, minerals, and water. Plant foods provide special value as they are the only source of fiber and, of course, contain a host of phytochemicals.

Energy in food is mainly supplied by carbohydrate (sugars and starches) and fats, and is measured in calories or Kilojoules. Very little protein is used for energy; our bodies prefer to harness it for growth, repair, and for the regulation of body processes. Vitamins and minerals help release energy from food for breathing, digesting food, brain, nerve and muscle function, heartbeat, temperature regulation, immunity, and physical activity. Fiber helps regulates blood glucose and cholesterol levels, and keeps the bowel and its bacteria healthy.

CARBOHYDRATE

Carbohydrate is the body's favorite fuel. The brain especially likes it and utilizes billions of glucose molecules

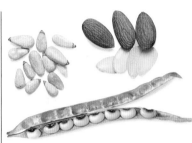

PROTEIN
Protein-rich plant foods are peas, beans, lentils, nuts, and seeds. Breads and other grains provide smaller amounts of protein.

every second. Digested carbohydrates are absorbed to top up blood glucose levels – used as an energy supply by our body cells. The body can also store small amounts of carbohydrate, called glycogen, in the muscles and liver, which is used as an immediate fuel for muscles and maintains blood glucose levels between meals.

Carbohydrate is divided into simple sugars – which include mono-saccharides e.g., glucose, fructose (or fruit sugar); disaccharides e.g., sucrose (or table sugar), lactose (or milk sugar); oligosaccharides e.g., fructo-oligosaccharides – and polysaccharides (or starch – plants' equivalent to our glycogen stores), and non-starch polysaccharides.

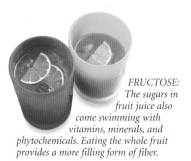

FRUCTOSE:
The sugars in fruit juice also come swimming with vitamins, minerals, and phytochemicals. Eating the whole fruit provides a more filling form of fiber.

FIBER AND INTESTINAL FLORA

Non-starch polysaccharides and fructo-oligosaccharides are both forms of fiber and structural parts of plants. Fiber differs from sugars and starch since it resists digestive enzymes. A form of starch known as resistant starch also escapes digestion. Fiber and resistant starch pass into the colon (large bowel) where they are broken down to different extents by the natural gut flora: the billions of bacteria that naturally dwell down there and work to help keep us healthy. They do this by acting as a barrier to potentially harmful bacteria, keeping the bowel contents moving, digesting and fermenting resistant starch and some fibers (the by-products of fermentation may help protect against cancer), stimulating the gut's immune system, and producing certain vitamins.

Some fibers, especially fructo-oligosaccharides, go one better and promote the growth of beneficial gut bacteria such as lactobacilli and bifidobacteria *(see p.98)*, which can be particularly helpful if the gut flora gets upset by diet, medication, illness, travel, or even stress.

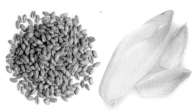

FIBER
Whole wheat is a good source of insoluble fiber and fructo-oligosaccharides, as is endive. Plant foods provide a variety of different fibers to optimize health benefits.

Nonstarch polysaccharide fiber can be divided into insoluble and soluble fiber. Insoluble fiber is found mainly in bran-based cereals, wholegrain flour, bread, and pasta, and most vegetables. It acts a bit like a sponge, soaking up and holding onto water in the bowel. The end result is a larger and softer bulk passing easily and regularly through the colon. A lack of insoluble fiber in the diet can lead to constipation.

Good amounts of soluble fiber are found in legumes, oats, barley, rye, and most fruit. It combines with water to make a gummy substance that slows digestion and absorption of food. This helps regulate the levels of glucose in our blood, makes us

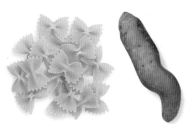

STARCHY CARBOHYDRATES
Bread, pasta, potatoes, cereal, noodles, rice, and grains provide starchy carbohydrates. Include wholegrain varieties in your diet for extra fiber, nutrients, and phytochemicals.

GLYCEMIC INDEX

The Glycemic Index (GI) is a ranking of foods ranging from 0-100 that reveals how quickly a food will affect a rise in blood glucose levels. The lower the GI, the more gradual the rise in blood glucose, and a more sustained and satisfying energy supply will result. Foods with a low GI are generally rich in soluble fiber and include oats, peas, beans, lentils, corn, pasta, rye, fruit, and granary breads, most fresh and dried fruit, noodles, granola, and bran cereals. Aim to make these foods a regular part of main meals.

feel fuller for longer after meals, and, as part of a healthy diet, can help manage cholesterol levels. Fiber also absorbs fluid; drink six to eight large glasses of fluid each day.

FATS

We all need some fat in our diet to stay healthy, and plant foods provide the healthiest types. Fat helps food taste good, provides energy, is part of cell membranes, supplies essential fatty acids, and promotes absorption of fat-soluble vitamins and carotenoid phytochemicals (p.72).

There are three main types of fats in foods: polyunsaturates, mono-unsaturates, and saturates. Saturated

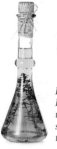

FATS
Polyunsaturates (e.g., in oil), mono-unsaturates (e.g., in avocado), and saturates (e.g., in coconut) are the three main fats in our diet.

fats are found mainly in animal foods such as fatty meat, cheese, and butter; with the exception of coconut and palm oil, plants are not important sources of saturated fat. Too many saturates (and trans fats, p.125) raise LDL cholesterol levels.

Good sources of monounsaturated fat include olive oil, rapeseed oil, avocados, and most nuts. Eaten in moderation, they have beneficial effects on blood cholesterol levels.

There are two families of polyunsaturated fats, each headed by a "parent" essential fatty acid: linoleic acid (omega-6 family); and alpha-linolenic acid (omega-3 family). These fatty acids are needed for growth, cell membranes, and to produce eicosanoids – chemical messengers that help regulate blood clotting, blood pressure, and immunity. Omega-3 fats are needed for early eye and brain development. In moderation, omega-6 fats help lower blood cholesterol levels.

The balance between these two families is important for their optimal function; we usually get plenty of omega-6 fats in our diet, so it is best to limit these and eat more omega-3s. Sources of omega-3 fats include rapeseed, linseed, soy and walnut oils, pumpkin seeds, whole-grains, walnuts, soy beans, sweet potatoes, green vegetables, and oily fish. Good sources of omega-6 fats include sunflower, safflower, and corn oils and margarine, grapeseed oil, sunflower and sesame seeds.

VITAMINS AND MINERALS

Vitamins and minerals are vital to life, and the only way we can get them naturally is from food. There are 13 different vitamins, which are all needed to help regulate body processes (see chart, right), and almost every action in the body needs the support of these vitamins. Some 15 minerals are known to be essential to humans. They can have a structural role – for example, calcium in bones – or help regulate fluid blood pressure and fluid balance. Minerals also form a part of enzymes, which help the metabolic processes.

	WHAT IT DOES	WHERE IT IS FOUND
VITAMIN C	Antioxidant; needed for healthy skin, bones, teeth, and gums; helps fight infection; aids iron absorption.	Citrus fruit and juice, berries, kiwifruit, melon, vegetables – especially peppers, greens, and potatoes.
VITAMIN E	Antioxidant that protects body cells and polyunsaturated fats. Works well with vitamin C.	Vegetable oils, nuts, seeds, wholegrains, and greens.
FOLATE	A B-vitamin, it helps reduce the risk of fetal spina bifida during pregnancy and helps lower the risk of heart disease. Needed for healthy blood and nerve function.	Wholegrain breads and cereals, greens, legumes, orange juice, variety meats, and food fortified with folic acid such as cereals, bread, and yeast extracts.

KEY MINERALS IN PLANT FOODS

	WHAT IT DOES	WHERE IT IS FOUND
MAGNESIUM	Allows the body to use energy from food. Works with calcium in muscle and nerve function. Gives bones rigidity.	Wholegrains, greens, nuts, legumes, seeds, fish, dried fruit, and bananas.
POTASSIUM	Helps regulate blood pressure, heartbeat, nerve and muscle function.	Juices, fruit, nuts, vegetables, legumes, wholegrains, meat, and dairy foods.
SELENIUM	Important part of antioxidant enzymes made in the body. Plays a role in cancer prevention, reproduction, and thyroid function.	Nuts, especially Brazil nuts, seaweed, wholegrains, fish, meat, and variety meats.
CALCIUM	Builds and maintains strong bones and teeth, helps prevent osteoporosis; needed for muscle and nerve function.	Milk, dairy foods, sardines, bread, legumes, nuts, greens, calcium-fortified soy milk, and juice.
IRON	Needed to form hemoglobin in red blood cells, which transport oxygen to body cells.	Wholegrains, fortified cereals, legumes, breads, greens, dried fruit, oily fish, and meat.

MAKING THE MOST OF PHYTOCHEMICALS

Enjoying a diet rich in plant foods helps protect our health, but including a wide variety of different-colored foods is also vital. As you delve more deeply into *Super Nutrients,* you'll discover exactly why.

The vibrant hues of Mediterranean foods give a tantalizing insight into the benefits of making meals colorful. The importance of such variety was reinforced by a study that showed women who ate a diet with a varied mix of vegetables had a 20 percent lower risk of colon cancer than women with a less varied intake. Perhaps not surprisingly, those who ate the most plant foods also had a 30 percent reduced risk of developing colon cancer compared to those who ate the least.

GETTING COLORFUL

The different colors of fruits and vegetables reflect the presence of different types of phytochemicals. Optimize your phytochemical mix by choosing from the selected super-foods for each color every day, as listed below. Deeper-colored fruit and vegetables tend to be richer in vitamins and minerals.

● **WHITE/YELLOW**

Onions, garlic, apples, pears, celery, lettuce, squash.

● **ORANGE/RED**

Citrus fruit, carrots, tomatoes, red peppers, apricots, melon, pumpkin.

● **RED/PURPLE**

Berries, cherries, plums, egg plant, dark grapes, prunes.

● **GREEN**

Spinach, broccoli, Brussels sprouts, kale, cabbage, watercress, parsley.

● **GREEN/BROWN**

Beans, lentils, pumpkin seeds, peanuts, walnuts, tea, chocolate.

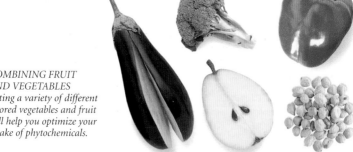

COMBINING FRUIT AND VEGETABLES
Eating a variety of different colored vegetables and fruit will help you optimize your intake of phytochemicals.

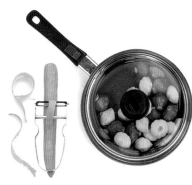

STORAGE AND COOKING
Protect the goodness in fruit and vegetables by storing and cooking them wisely. Prepare vegetables as near to the time of cooking as possible to retain their nutrients.

PROTECTING NUTRIENTS

Research into the effects of storage and cooking on phytochemicals is still in its infancy, but heat, light, and air can destroy sensitive vitamins, while minerals (and some phytochemicals) can leach into cooking water *(see also Part Two)*.

BUYING

Avoid wilted, bruised, or blemished produce; look for strong, bright colors. Buy regularly, store well, and eat soon after purchase – sensitive vitamin C and folic acid start to dwindle as soon as the produce has been picked.

STORING

Fresh produce stays crisper and its vitamins last longer stored in the refrigerator. Or keep in a cool, dark, well-ventilated place and try to consume within two to three days.

Take care not to pile too many soft fruits in a fruit basket; they may quickly bruise and go bad. Store seeds in the fridge in an airtight container. Wholewheat flour and other wholegrains are also best stored this way to reduce the risk of rancidity (oxygen can react with the unsaturated fats they contain). Dried beans and lentils store well in an airtight container in a cool place.

PREPARING AND COOKING

Raw fruits and vegetables give you the most nutrition per mouthful; wash, scrub, or peel thinly and enjoy the crunch. Avoid presoaking, unnecessary peeling and slicing, keeping warm, or reheating vegetables, and do not add bicarbonate of soda to preserve color – it destroys vitamins.

Microwave, steam, pressure cook, stir fry, or boil fruit and vegetables in a minimum of cooking water; the quicker the method, the better. Cook until just tender. Soak and cook raw legumes according to directions; undercooked legumes may be toxic *(see p.112)*.

ANTIOXIDANT SCALE

ORAC (oxygen radical absorbance capacity) units are a method of measuring the antioxidant capacity of fruit and vegetables. Foods are ranked according to their potential to mop up oxygen-free radicals. Choosing foods with high ORAC levels gives a special boost. Cocoa powder, then green tea, ranks highest per 4oz.; prunes and raisins rank high, too, but these are all dried foods and are much more concentrated (and eaten in smaller amounts) than fresh fruit and vegetables.

Top 10 ORAC scores per 4oz. fresh produce: blueberries, blackberries, garlic, kale, strawberries, spinach, Brussels sprouts, plums, alfalfa sprouts, broccoli.

FUNCTIONAL, GM, & ORGANIC FOODS

Advancements in food technology, often using phytochemicals, are progressing at a rapid pace. Amid designer functional foods and GM foods, organic food is also flourishing.

Japan launched the "nutraceutical" or functional food fashion in the late '80s, and today it has an industry worth more than two billion dollars. In the West there is no legal definition of a functional food, but nutritionists have defined it as a food ingredient containing health-promoting benefits and/or disease-preventing properties over and above its usual nutritional value.

FUNCTIONAL FOODS

There are two categories of functional foods: foods that have well-known ingredients added to them – for example, calcium in orange juice, omega-3 fats in margarine or eggs, phytoestrogen-rich linseeds and soy flour in bread *(p.48)*; and foods with newly identified or "novel" ingredients – for example, cholesterol-lowering plant stanol esters or sterols in margarines, or "live" bacteria in yogurt and drinks *(probiotics, p.98)*. Then there are "interesting" alternatives, such as St John's wort in chips or soup!

Without tight regulation, there is great scope for misleading consumers with exaggerated claims about health benefits or, at worst, providing unsafe foods. So far, regulation has been on a largely voluntary basis backed up by standard food laws concerning food labeling and health claims. By making sure that information about a functional food is accurate and supported by scientific research, we, as consumers, can make more informed choices.

Some functional foods may well have positive health effects, but they are not an instant answer to health. Proven, specific benefits of certain foods means that they will be more beneficial for some people than others. Sometimes the "carrier" food is loaded with fat, sugar, or salt

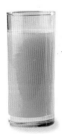

ORANGE JUICE
Drinks such as fruit juice may have added vitamins and minerals.

MARGARINE
Margarine can be a vehicle for omega 3 fats or cholesterol-lowering ingredients.

(think phytochemical-enriched candy and chips!). There is also the danger that functional foods could blur the boundaries between food groups and confuse people about the basis of nutrition recommen-dations (*p.18*). Eating a varied and balanced diet is still the mainstay of good nutrition, and functional foods are not intended to be a replacement.

GM FOODS

Genetic engineering is a technique used to copy and transfer genes from one plant, animal, or micro-organism to another, or to alter genetic material (DNA) and achieve desired changes in its characteristics – for example, increase plant pest resistance, improve nutrient content or flavor, or give higher yields. There has been much debate about the long-term effects of GM foods on our health and on the environment, as well as ethical and labeling issues. Governments, scientists, farmers, the food industry, and consumers must work together to guarantee safe, beneficial use and progression of any GM technology.

ORGANIC FOOD

Organic plant food is produce that has been grown without fertilizers or pesticides and in a way that works with natural systems rather than dominating them, so minimizing damage to the environment and wildlife. Genetic modification technology or GM ingredients are not permitted. Production of organic food is legally regulated, and growers must be registered with official bodies. Whether or not to eat organic foods really boils down to personal choice. For people who wish to support the ecological benefits of organic farming, minimize any exposure to pesticides, and avoid GM produce, organic foods are the best choice. But cost may be an issue, and there is currently no clear evidence that organic food is healthier, better-tasting, or more nutritious than conventionally produced plant foods. However, organic produce tends to contain less water, so some foods may have a higher concentration of nutrients by weight.

EXAMPLES OF GM FOODS

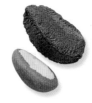

BRAZIL NUTS
A gene from Brazil nuts transferred to soy beans carried the nut's allergens. The project was stopped.

SOY BEANS
Currently in use are GM soy beans that are resistant to a universal weedkiller, reducing the need for weed-killers on crops.

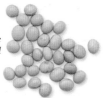

WHITE RICE
GM betacarotene-rich rice is being developed to improve vitamin-A deficiency in develop-ing countries.

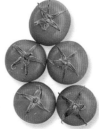

TOMATOES
GM tomato purée claims improved flavor, color, and cost. GM tomatoes with more carotenoids are being developed.

SUPPLEMENTS AND NUTRITION RESEARCH

Popping a pill supplement at meals may seem like an easy answer to getting your daily phytochemical fix. But good nutrition isn't that simple, and taking too much of a good thing may do more harm than good.

More and more phytochemical supplements are now available from stores, magazines, and the internet. The most popular so far include carotenoids, quercetin, isoflavones, garlic, artichoke or red wine extracts, plant enzymes, and fructo-oligosaccharides.

UNDERSTANDING NUTRITION RESEARCH

As you will discover in Part Two, each phytochemical has plausible biological mechanisms as to why it could potentially help our health. But more research is needed to know whether taking phytochemical supplements will actually be helpful, and if so what are safe and effective doses and who might benefit most.

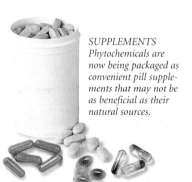

SUPPLEMENTS
Phytochemicals are now being packaged as convenient pill supplements that may not be as beneficial as their natural sources.

Safety is paramount, since a large study of male smokers taking high daily doses (30mg) of betacarotene had to be stopped as the risk of these men getting lung cancer actually increased (researchers were hoping to decrease it). And at very high doses, phytochemicals or vitamins that usually act as antioxidants may instead act as potentially damaging pro-oxidants (also see pp.108-109).

The health supplement industry as a whole is set for better regulation, with more product information to be supplied to consumers. Ongoing research could mean that one day some supplements will be prescribed to help prevent or treat medical conditions. Meanwhile, be wary of a supplement that makes claims which aren't supported by expert scientific evidence, and if you are on medication, get advice from your doctor before taking supplements. Remember, too, that food provides phytochemicals and nutrients in a ready packaged and delicious form.

Nutrition research is an evolutionary process. Even at its best, it can never prove outright that a certain diet or food will protect against or treat a particular problem since there are so many other health-related lifestyle factors to consider. Phytochemical research is helping us make sense of trends and associations from studies of different populations. But to be clearer about the way phytochemicals can reduce disease risk and benefit health, more controlled human intervention trials are needed.

MAIN TYPES OF NUTRITION RESEARCH

◆ Epidemiological or population studies: these help researchers narrow down a list of potential causes by showing possible associations between dietary or environmental factors and a particular disease. There are a number of different types, and while none can prove cause and effect – researchers can control for some factors that may contribute to a disease but not all – they help progress research by initiating further studies.

◆ Basic research: experiments carried out under controlled laboratory conditions, which may be done in a test tube, with animals, or using human or animal cells or tissues. They tell us what happens inside cells, but not about what actually happens when we eat and digest foods.

◆ Intervention or clinical trials: these involve people who follow a specific regime and include at least one "treatment" group and "control" group, which receive either an inactive (placebo) or existing treatment.

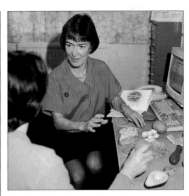

NUTRITIONAL RESEARCH
Intervention trials can have direct implications for human health. People are randomly assigned to treatment or control groups to help account for known and unknown dietary and environmental factors.

More trials are needed to help us fully understand phytochemicals but ethics, safety, time, and cost must also be considered.

Two terms frequently used in scientific studies are: "association" – there may be a connection that cannot be explained by coincidence but is not proven; and "significant" – unlikely that the results would have been obtained if there is no real effect or association.

Conclusions cannot be drawn from single studies; additional studies answer some questions but pose others. Results from all these different studies are relevant, and also necessary, to help make judgments about the effects of diet, individual foods, and dietary supplements on health. Meanwhile, you can be confident that there is a large and ever-increasing body of evidence to show that a varied, plant food-rich diet, combined with an active, tobacco-free lifestyle, will help us to live long and healthy lives.

ASSESS YOUR PHYTO-CHEMICAL INTAKE

Find out how your fruit and vegetable intake fares by answering this quick questionnaire. If you can't remember what you usually eat, keep a food record for a few days and see how it measures up.

QUESTIONNAIRE

	A	B	C
1. Do you always start the day with breakfast?	○	○	○
2. Do you eat regular meals through the day and include a variety of foods from the five food groups?	○	○	○
3. Do you have a portion of some type of fruit or vegetable with each meal?	○	○	○
4. Do you eat at least five portions of fruit and vegetables every day?	○	○	○
5. Do you include a portion of citrus fruit such as oranges, grapefruit, or satsumas (two satsumas counts as a portion of fruit) on a daily basis?	○	○	○

YOUR SCORE   A - USUALLY   B - OCCASIONALLY   C - RARELY

Check how your diet measures up to the optimal intakes of different plant foods and use the results, and the information throughout *Super Nutrients*, to help you achieve a healthy diet that suits your tastes and lifestyle. You don't have to get a perfect score to benefit from phytochemical-rich plant foods; any changes you can make to insure there are some "As" in your score is great progress!

For details of what constitutes a serving or portion and balanced diets, see pp.18-19. For more information about the benefits of following the recommendations from this quiz, see pp.20-23.

• **MAINLY AS**
Well done. Your diet is brimming with a wide variety of different and colorful plant foods. If you scored A on question 2, it is also well balanced. Both variety and quantity are important as this way you get an optimal mix of nutrients and phytochemicals. Research suggests that the more varied your plant food intake, the more protective your diet may be against chronic diseases. The good super-nutrient mix you'll get helps you fight infections and keep up energy levels, too. A plant food-rich diet can also help you stay in shape.

		A	B	C
6	Do you include a portion of green vegetables such as broccoli, cabbage, dark green lettuce, spinach, or asparagus on a daily basis?	○	○	○
7	Do you include a portion of red and/or orange fruit and vegetables such as tomatoes, red peppers, mangoes, pumpkin, carrots, and apricots on a daily basis?	○	○	○
8	Do you include a serving of legumes such as peas, lentils, or beans (includes canned beans) four or more times a week?	○	○	○
9	Do you eat 1oz (28g) of nuts, seeds, or nut butters four or more times a week?	○	○	○
10	Do you eat six or more servings of starchy food such as breakfast cereal, bread, pasta, potatoes, noodles, and rice each day?	○	○	○
11	Do three servings of these starchy foods comprise wholegrain types, for example, wholemeal or rye bread, wholegrain cereal, oats, brown rice, or wholewheat pasta?	○	○	○
12	Do you use oils and fats rich in monounsaturated or polyunsaturated fats rather than saturated or trans fat (such as lard, butter, and hard margarines) for baking, frying, and spreading?	○	○	○

• **MAINLY BS**

Although you are currently eating a diet that provides a reasonable mix of plant foods and their bounty of nutrients and phytochemicals, you can still boost the benefits more. Look back to see where you can make changes; perhaps start in areas where you scored a C. Then move on to the Bs. Choose one at a time, and plan simple ways to change. For example, if you do not currently eat legumes, have beans on toast, serve peas or beans as a side vegetable, or add beans or lentils to soups, salads, and casseroles.

• **MAINLY CS**

You are eating a diet that is relatively low in plant foods and the rich supply of beneficial nutrients and phytochemicals they provide. To improve your diet, make changes step by step. For example, if like most people you eat about three portions of fruit and vegetables daily, try having four, then move up to five portions a day. When you feel comfortable with that, focus on having a wide variety each day. Start with changes you'll find easiest to make, and remember, small changes add to up make a big difference.

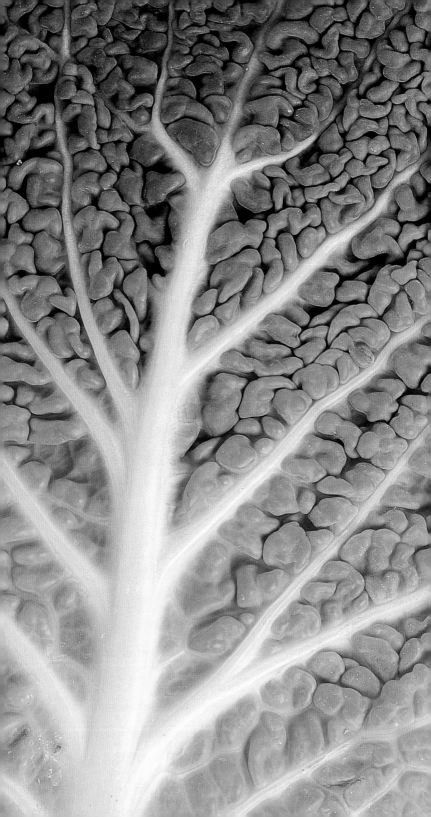

Part Two

Welcome to a photographic guide to 30

phytochemicals, highlighted by 66 different food

sources. Each phytochemical has a personal

profile outlining its key benefits as supported by

current scientific research, and information on

how to maximize its goodness.

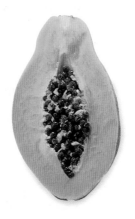

GUIDE TO PHENOLIC COMPOUNDS

Phenolic compounds are the largest category of phyto-chemicals and occur naturally in fruit, vegetables, herbs, nuts, seeds, flowers, and bark. Plants produce these phytochemicals to protect their own health, longevity, and reproduction.

Phenolic compounds (also referred to as phenolics, or polyphenols) first interested nutritionists because of their effects on the absorption of nutrients. This was superseded by the discovery that phenolics act as powerful antioxidants and anti-cancer agents, which means that they have the potential to protect our health, too.

FLAVONOIDS

Flavonoids are the largest category of phenolic compounds and are responsible for the deep blue color of delphiniums, the bold "bite" of grapefruit, the vivid red blush of fresh cherries, and the refreshing astringency of a cup of tea.

Over 4,000 different types of flavonoids have been identified, and they are widespread throughout plant foods. They were first discovered by a Hungarian scientist in 1936 in the white rind of citrus fruits, and initially earned the name vitamin P (for "permeability"), due to their beneficial role in keeping blood vessels healthy. Only a relatively small number of plant species have had their flavonoid content carefully investigated so far, but enough is now known to give some guidance about how to make the most of flavonoids.

BENEFICIAL PROPERTIES

Two examples of foods containing beneficial flavonoids are the onion and apple. They are not rich in high–profile nutrients such as vitamin C and folate, so until the advent of flavonoid research their nutritional profile was relatively low. Now they are high up on the "good for your heart" league, and a must for the health-conscious.

Tea and wine are also of special interest because they too are strongly linked to heart health and rich in flavonoids (which are well absorbed by the body), yet don't contain the classic antioxidants – namely, vitamins C and E (see p.23). This helps make the case that flavonoids are responsible for much of their benefit. In fact, flavonoids have been shown to be more potent antioxidants than vitamins C and E, and can protect the body from free radical attack. They also make vitamin C work more effectively.

Flavonoids are extraordinarily active. When tested in laboratory settings they display a range of biological effects, including antiinflammatory, anticancer, antiviral, antibacterial, and blood vessel relaxing abilities. By acting as antioxidants, they inhibit the oxidation of "bad" LDL cholesterol and cell membranes. They seem to affect platelet aggregation (or "stickiness") blood vessels, and inflammation by influencing specific enzyme actions in the body.

FLAVONOID ABSORPTION

Research is now focused on how flavonoids are absorbed and how active they are in the body. Gut flora (bacteria that naturally live in the large intestine) actually change the structure of flavonoids to maximize their absorption, so differences in people's gut flora can mean differences in absorption. A fiber-rich, high carbohydrate diet can promote a healthy balance of gut flora (see pp.20–21), which in turn may optimize flavonoid absorption. Once absorbed, a flavonoid's structure changes again and is then ready to get to work and also interact with nutrients and other phytochemicals.

HEALTH LINKS

Despite the need for further clarification about how flavonoids work in the body, population studies clearly point to links between a high intake of flavonoid-rich foods – fruit, vegetables, tea, red wine – and a reduced risk of heart disease and stroke. While flavonoids have been shown to have anticancer actions in laboratory settings, the population evidence for cancer protection is less clear.

Find out more about some of the main flavonoids and their sources on the following pages. Here is a quick guide to flavonoid-rich foods:

◆ ANTHOCYANINS
Cherries, eggplant, cranberries, blueberries, blackberries, raspberries, strawberries, black grapes, radishes, blackcurrants, red wine, elderberries.

◆ FLAVONES: LUTEOLIN, APIGENIN
Celery, olives, parsley, lemons, red peppers, artichokes, oranges, chili peppers.

◆ FLAVANOLS: CATECHINS
Green tea, black tea, cocoa and chocolate, red and white wine, pears, apples.

◆ FLAVONOLS: QUERCETIN, RUTIN
Onions, apples, lettuce (especially Lollo Rosso), kale, wine, olives, potatoes, leeks, tea, tomatoes (especially cherry tomatoes), endive, broccoli, buckwheat, berries, peas, cabbage, parsley, cauliflower, green beans, oats, Brussels sprouts.

◆ FLAVANONES: NARINGENIN, HESPERIDIN
Citrus fruit and peel – of orange, grapefruit, lemon, lime, tangerines, satsumas, mandarins and kumquats – prunes, cashew nuts.

◆ ISOFLAVONES
See p.48

CHERRY

Offers anti-inflammatory benefits ◆ May
promote heart health ◆ Has antioxidant effects

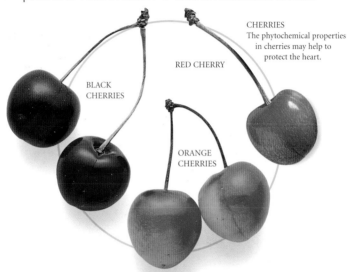

CHERRIES
The phytochemical properties
in cherries may help to
protect the heart.

RED CHERRY

BLACK
CHERRIES

ORANGE
CHERRIES

MAXIMIZING THE BENEFITS

Enjoy your cherries fresh; cooking will leach some anthocyanins into the cooking water. Green stalks are a sign of freshness, and to preserve vitamin C, the cherries should be stored in the refrigerator. Some people are allergic to a specific protein in cherries.

HOW MUCH TO EAT

An average portion of 10 cherries, containing pits, weighs 2oz. Eat a handful as a snack, or bake or stew and freeze; there is no need to remove the stones or blanch first.

KEY BENEFITS

The phytochemical anthocyanin gives cherries their red, purple, or black color. It is the most important color pigment in flower and fruit plants, and extracts are used for food coloring. Anthocyanin has strong antioxidant and anti-inflammatory effects.

● HEART DISEASE

Laboratory studies on anthocyanin show antioxidant effects that might help prevent the build-up of fatty deposits in the arteries (atherosclerosis). Other studies show the anti-inflammatory benefits of anthocyanins that may also help to protect the heart.

● CANCER

A study on the effects of anthocyanins on colon cancer cells showed no beneficial effect inside cells, but did show a strong potential for neutralizing nitrogen-containing free radicals in the blood–stream or colon. This might help protect against stomach and colon cancer.

CHERRY: OTHER PHYTOCHEMICALS

OTHER FLAVONOIDS	pp.34–35
PHENOLIC ACIDS	pp.56–57
MONOTERPENES	p.102

NUTRITIONAL VALUES
Quantities per 4oz.

CALORIES	39
FIBER	1g
POTASSIUM	170mg
VITAMIN C	9mg

EGGPLANT

Blocks formation of free radicals ◆ May help reduce cholesterol levels ◆ Source of folic acid and potassium

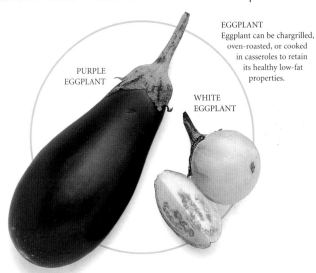

EGGPLANT
Eggplant can be chargrilled, oven-roasted, or cooked in casseroles to retain its healthy low-fat properties.

PURPLE EGGPLANT

WHITE EGGPLANT

MAXIMIZING THE BENEFITS

Eggplant is best eaten cooked. Larger eggplants contain bitter juices, which can be drawn out by slicing and salting the eggplant. After 20-30 minutes rinse and wipe dry. Do this just before cooking to prevent flesh discoloration.

HOW MUCH TO EAT

Half an eggplant weighs 6oz. It is a low-fat vegetable but absorbs copious amounts of fat when fried. Limit this by drawing out the juices *(above)* or using low-fat cooking methods.

KEY BENEFITS

A type of anthocyanin called nasuin is responsible for the glossy purple of eggplant skin; white eggplants contain other types of flavonoids. Nasuin is a potent antioxidant. Originating from India, the eggplant is a colorful staple of the heart-healthy diets of Asia, the Middle East, and the Mediterranean, and is now popular worldwide.

● **PROTECTS AGAINST CELL DAMAGE**
Laboratory studies reveal that nasuin extracted from eggplant skin works as an antioxidant by blocking the formation of free radicals. This helps protect against damage to cell membranes and "bad" LDL cholesterol, reducing the risk of atherosclerosis.

● **CHOLESTEROL LEVELS**
In animal studies, daily quantities of eggplant juice have been shown to reduce cholesterol levels and promote the health of blood vessels.

EGGPLANT: OTHER PHYTOCHEMICALS

| PHENOLIC ACIDS pp.56–57 |
| PHYTOSTEROLS p.97 |
| GLYKOALKALOIDS p.111 |

NUTRITIONAL VALUES
Quantities per 4oz. (raw)

CALORIES	15
FIBER	2g
POTASSIUM	210mg
FOLATE	18mcg

CHOCOLATE & COCOA

Has antioxidant effects ◆ May benefit

the heart ◆ Source of iron and potassium

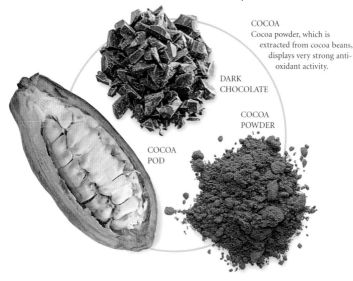

COCOA
Cocoa powder, which is
extracted from cocoa beans,
displays very strong antioxidant activity.

DARK
CHOCOLATE

COCOA
POWDER

COCOA
POD

MAXIMIZING THE BENEFITS

Choose unsweetened or dark chocolate with high cocoa solids (ideally 70%) for the highest catechin content. It is also a source of iron, copper , and magnesium; white and milk chocolate provide more calcium.

HOW MUCH TO EAT

2oz. of milk chocolate is reported to have a similar level of phenolic antioxidants as a glass of red wine (p.68). It is also high in fat and sugar, and so should be eaten in moderation and not in place of fruit and vegetables.

KEY BENEFITS

Flavanols, also known as catechins, are the most prominent phytochemical in cocoa beans. Complex catechin-based antioxidants (procyanidins) are formed during the process of making chocolate from cocoa powder, which adds to its unique flavor.

● **HEART HEALTH**
Laboratory and human studies show that consuming flavanol-rich cocoa can inhibit platelet activation and aggregation (*see also p.125*). Researchers suggest that these beneficial effects are due to a very mild "aspirin-like" effect from flavanol-based procyanidins

(aspirin is known for its benefits on circulation).

● **ANTIOXIDANT EFFECTS**
A recent trial in the U.S. showed that the "bad" cholesterol of people who consumed cocoa powder and chocolate daily had more protection from oxidation (oxidized LDL triggers atherosclerosis).

DARK CHOCOLATE: OTHER PHYTOCHEMICALS

NUTRITIONAL VALUES
Quantities per 4oz.

CALORIES	510
FIBER	2.5g
MAGNESIUM	89mg

GREEN TEA

May reduce the risk of heart disease and stroke

Has anticancer effects ◆ Helps fight tooth decay

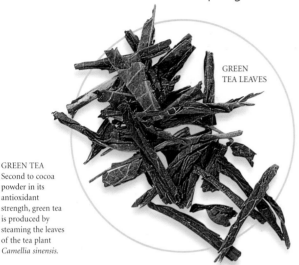

GREEN
TEA LEAVES

GREEN TEA
Second to cocoa
powder in its
antioxidant
strength, green tea
is produced by
steaming the leaves
of the tea plant
Camellia sinensis.

MAXIMIZING THE BENEFITS

The flavanols in green tea are very soluble and are absorbed well by the body. Allow it to brew for at least a minute for maximum release of flavonoids in the hot liquid.

HOW MUCH TO DRINK

A Dutch study revealed that just one cup of green tea (1tsp. in 1¼c. water) led to a significant increase in antioxidant activity in the blood of volunteers (and more activity than from black tea). Four to five cups may give optimal benefits.

KEY BENEFITS

Epicatechin flavanols, the main phytochemicals in green tea, have been shown to have antioxidant, anti-thrombotic, antibacterial, antiviral, anticancer, and immune system regulating effects.

● HEART DISEASE

A Japanese study showed that drinking green tea regularly may significantly lower cholesterol levels. This may be explained partly by flavanols' ability to inhibit cholesterol absorption into the body.

● CANCERS

A Chinese study indicated a link between drinking green tea and a reduced incidence of cancer of the esophagus and stomach. An animal study found that drinking green tea inhibited the development of blood vessels needed to support the growth of cancerous tumors.

● TOOTH DECAY

Flavanols may protect against tooth decay by inhibiting the bacterial activities that lead to a buildup of plaque.

GREEN TEA: OTHER PHYTOCHEMICALS

| OTHER FLAVONOIDS | pp.34–35 |
| PHENOLIC ACIDS | pp.56–57 |

NUTRITIONAL VALUES
Quantities per 4oz.

| CALORIES | Negligible |
| FIBER | Negligible |

BLACK TEA

Linked to good bone health ◆ Has anticancer effects

May help reduce the risk of heart disease and stroke

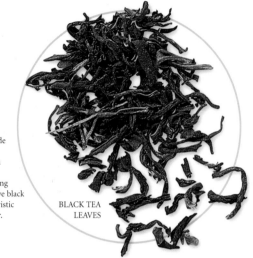

BLACK TEA
Black tea is made
by fermenting
leaves of the tea
plant *Camellia
sinensis*. Its strong
antioxidants give black
tea its characteristic
color and flavor.

BLACK TEA
LEAVES

MAXIMIZING THE BENEFITS

Brew tea for at least a minute to maximize the release of flavanols. Adding milk does not affect absorption. The phenolic compounds in tea can reduce iron absorption from non-meat foods, so do not drink tea with every meal. The fluorine in tea helps protect against tooth decay.

HOW MUCH TO DRINK

Positive health benefits have been associated with drinking 1–5 cups of black tea, or decaffeinated black tea, daily.

KEY BENEFITS

Flavanols are the main phytochemicals in black tea. Simple flavanols are transformed into complex flavanols (thearubigens and theaflavins) during the fermentation process.

● **BONE HEALTH**
A study of 1,256 women in Britain aged 65 to 76 found that regular tea drinkers had significantly stronger bones than non-tea drinkers, suggesting that tea flavonoids may influence bone health.

● **CANCER**
A study of 35,369 post-menopausal women in the U.S. indicated that those who drank two or more cups of black tea daily had 40-70 percent lower rates of digestive and urinary tract cancers compared to those who rarely drank tea.

● **HEART DISEASE**
A number of population studies link high flavonoid intakes, especially from regular tea drinking, with a reduced risk of heart disease and stroke.

BLACK TEA: OTHER PHYTOCHEMICALS

OTHER FLAVONOIDS	pp.34–35
PHENOLIC ACIDS	pp.56–57
XANTHINE ALKALOIDS	p.105

NUTRITIONAL VALUES
per cup (no milk)

CALORIES	Negligible
FIBER	Negligible
FLUORIDE	1mg

APPLE

Has anticancer effects ◆ Helps protect
against stroke ◆ Benefits bowel function

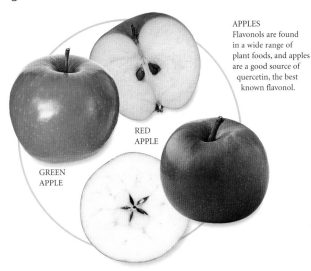

APPLES
Flavonols are found
in a wide range of
plant foods, and apples
are a good source of
quercetin, the best
known flavonol.

RED
APPLE

GREEN
APPLE

MAXIMIZING THE BENEFITS

Flavonols, especially quercetin, are well absorbed by the body. Eating fresh apples will maximize flavonol intake. Stewing can reduce levels by up to 70% as flavonols leach into cooking water, so eat the cooking juice, too. Limit peeling as flavonols concentrate near and in fruit skins.

HOW MUCH TO EAT

A medium apple weighs 4oz. (no core); an average glass of juice is 5oz. Eat apples as snacks, in fruit salads, grated on cereal, as juice, baked, or stewed.

KEY BENEFITS

The flavonol quercetin, which is found in apples, is one of the most potent antioxidants of flavonoids. Quercetin also has anti-inflammatory and anticancer actions.

● **LUNG CANCER**
A 24-year study of 10,000 Finnish people found that, after taking other diet and lifestyle factors into consideration, there was a strong association between eating plenty of apples and a reduced risk of developing lung cancer.

● **STROKE**
An investigation into the link between the quercetin intake of 9,200 Finnish adults, and the subsequent incidence of stroke over the following 28 years, revealed that while there was no direct association between quercetin intake per se, regular apple eaters had a 59 percent lower risk of stroke – reinforcing the importance of eating whole foods rather than separate supplements.

APPLES: OTHER PHYTOCHEMICALS

OTHER FLAVONOIDS pp.34–35

PHENOLIC ACIDS pp.56–57

CONDENSED TANNINS pp.67–68

NUTRITIONAL VALUES
Quantities per 4oz.

CALORIES	47
FIBER	1.8g
POTASSIUM	120mg

ONION

Linked to a reduced risk of heart disease

Has anti-inflammatory and anticancer effects

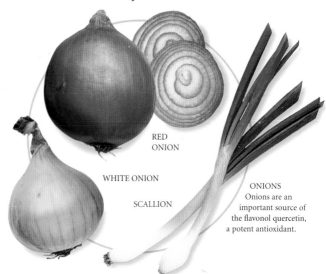

RED ONION

WHITE ONION

SCALLION

ONIONS
Onions are an important source of the flavonol quercetin, a potent antioxidant.

MAXIMIZING INTAKE

The highest concentration of quercetin is found in red, and then yellow onions; white onions contain none. Pan frying will not reduce the quercetin content, but cooking in water will. Animal studies suggest raw onion juice may have beneficial effects on the body's circulation.

HOW MUCH TO EAT

A small onion weighs 3oz., a thick slice 1oz. Slice raw into sandwich fillings or salads, roast, or add to pizzas, gravy, soups, pasta sources, curries, and casseroles.

KEY BENEFITS

Laboratory studies show that quercetin protects against free radical damage to "bad" LDL cholesterol. It also inhibits platelet aggregation, (but no similar effects resulted from eating onions).

● **HEART DISEASE**
Flavonol intakes might be linked to a reduced risk of heart disease. Onions were found to be one of the most important sources of flavonols in relevant studies conducted in the U.S., Finland, former Yugoslavia, and Greece.

● **ARTHRITIS**
Foods rich in antioxidants such as onions are recom-mended for people with arthritis. In laboratory studies, quercetin's anti-oxidant effects showed the potential to reduce the inflammation associated with rheumatoid arthritis.

● **CANCER**
Onions have been linked to a reduced risk of stomach cancer (see p.89).

ONION: OTHER PHYTOCHEMICALS

OTHER FLAVONOIDS pp.34–35

ALLIUM COMPOUNDS pp.88–89

FRUCTO-OLIGOSACCHARIDES pp.98–99

NUTRITIONAL VALUES
Quantities per 4oz.

CALORIES	36
FIBER	1.4g
POTASSIUM	160mg

LOLLO ROSSO LETTUCE

Has anticancer effects ◆ Helps keep bones strong

Good source of folate and potassium

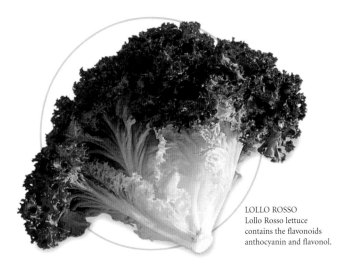

LOLLO ROSSO
Lollo Rosso lettuce
contains the flavonoids
anthocyanin and flavonol.

MAXIMIZING INTAKE

Choose Lollo Rosso for its superior flavonol content (its distinctive red ruffle is due to anthocyanins). Other types of lettuce are richer in different phytochemicals and nutrients, so a mixed-leaf salad is best.

HOW MUCH TO EAT

Four large leaves weigh about 3oz. Rinse to remove any surface pesticides or soil. Eat regularly by establishing the habit of including a salad as part of the main meal. Also use in sandwiches and as part of a generous garnish.

KEY BENEFITS

Lollo Rosso is ten times richer in the flavanol quercetin than iceberg lettuce, giving it strong antioxidant properties.

● CANCER

More than 60 studies have indicated cancer protection from green vegetables such as lettuce. Flavonols, alongside other nutrients and phytochemicals such as lutein (pp.80–81), will contribute to this effect.

● BONE HEALTH

A study on 72,327 women in the U.S., and their risk of breaking a hip in the following ten years, found that those who ate lettuce at least once a day had half the risk compared to those who ate one or no servings a week. High vitamin K intakes (of which Lollo Rosso lettuce is a good source) were also linked to decreased fracture risk. Other studies have suggested an association between bone strength and fruit and vegetable or flavonoid intake (see p.38).

LOLLO ROSSO: OTHER PHYTOCHEMICALS

OTHER FLAVONOIDS	pp.34–35
PHENOLIC ACIDS	pp.56–57
CAROTENOIDS	pp.72–73

NUTRITIONAL VALUES
Approximate values per 4oz.

CALORIES	16
FIBER	1.2g
FOLATE	50mcg
POTASSIUM	220mg

CELERY

May benefit blood pressure ◆ Has anti-inflammatory effects

A good source of potassium

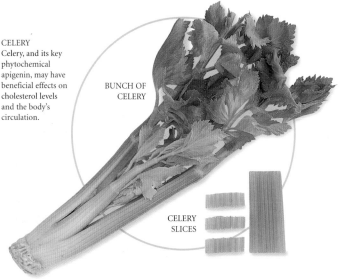

CELERY
Celery, and its key phytochemical apigenin, may have beneficial effects on cholesterol levels and the body's circulation.

BUNCH OF CELERY

CELERY SLICES

MAXIMIZING THE BENEFITS

Maximize the flavone content of celery by eating it raw, or use the cooking water in soups and gravy. The darker green sticks are higher in carotenoids (pp.72-73). Celery can accumulate high levels of nitrate from the soil, so avoid eating large amounts often (p.109).

HOW MUCH TO EAT

Three-four sticks weigh 4–6oz. Eating this amount regularly may be beneficial and not problematic in terms of nitrates. Eat raw or steam, or add to soups and casseroles.

KEY BENEFITS

The flavone apigenin is a key phytochemical in celery. Like all flavonoids it has antioxidant properties.

● **BLOOD PRESSURE**
Animal studies reveal that apigenin can relax blood vessels (which may benefit blood pressure) and also that 3-n-butyl phthalide (another phytochemical in celery, which gives it its distinctive smell) has a blood pressure lowering effect. Celery is a good source of potassium, which can also benefit blood pressure.

● **BOWEL CANCER**
A study assessing the role of diet in the development of colon cancer in China found a strong protective effect from vegetable intake, in particular from celery, chives, and leafy green vegetables.

● **INFLAMMATION**
Apigenin and celery extracts have both been shown to have anti-inflammatory properties.

CELERY: OTHER PHYTOCHEMICALS

OTHER FLAVONOIDS	pp.34–35
CAROTENOIDS	pp.72–73
COUMARINS	p.71

NUTRITIONAL VALUES
Quantities per 4oz.

CALORIES	7
FIBER	1.1g
POTASSIUM	320mg
FOLATE	16mcg

OLIVE & OLIVE OIL

Linked to a reduced risk of breast cancer ◆ Delays effects of aging ◆ Helps protect against rheumatoid arthritis

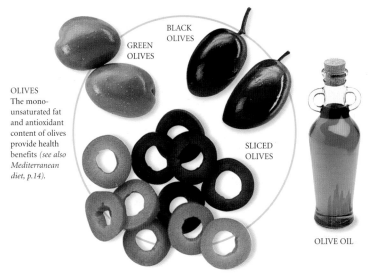

BLACK OLIVES

GREEN OLIVES

OLIVES
The mono-unsaturated fat and antioxidant content of olives provide health benefits *(see also Mediterranean diet, p.14).*

SLICED OLIVES

OLIVE OIL

MAXIMIZING THE BENEFITS

Virgin olive oil is "pressed" from olives; "extra virgin" olive oil is richest in phenolic compounds. Raw olives are bitter due to a phenolic compound, oleuropein, and are made edible by being pickled or marinaded in salt or oil.

HOW MUCH TO EAT

One olive (no stone) weighs ⅒oz. Olives are high in salt, so people with high blood pressure should moderate their intake. Use olive oil (which is high in calories) as a dressing and in cooking.

KEY BENEFITS

Flavones are one of the phenolic phytochemicals in olives. Olive oil contains a range of other phenolics *(see p.34).* Phenolics, along with vitamin E, give the olive, and olive oil, its well-known antioxidant power.

● HEART HEALTH
Olive oil is rich in mono-unsaturated fats, which have beneficial effects on the body's cholesterol levels. Human studies investigating diets rich in olive oil also show blood pressure-lowering and anti-blood clotting effects. All benefit health and help explain the longevity of people who enjoy a Mediterranean diet.

● CANCER
Population studies link diets high in monoun-saturated fat and/or olive oil with a reduced risk of breast cancer.

● MEMORY
A Mediterranean diet high in extra virgin olive oil might help to protect against age-related decline in mental function.

OLIVES: OTHER PHYTOCHEMICALS

OTHER FLAVONOIDS	pp.34–35
PHENOLIC ACIDS	pp.56–57
PHYTOSTEROLS	p.97

NUTRITIONAL VALUES
per 4oz. (no pit, in brine)

CALORIES	103
FIBER	2.9g
VITAMIN E	2mg

ORANGE

Helps lower cholesterol levels ◆ Has anticancer effects

Good source of vitamin C and folic acid

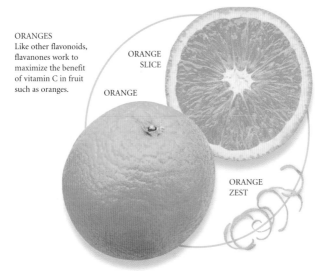

ORANGES
Like other flavonoids, flavanones work to maximize the benefit of vitamin C in fruit such as oranges.

ORANGE SLICE

ORANGE

ORANGE ZEST

MAXIMIZING THE BENEFITS

Eat oranges fresh to maximize flavanone, vitamin C, and folate benefits. The pith and membranes are rich sources of flavanones and pectin. The rind is also a source of phyto-chemicals. They are best stored in a refrigerator.

HOW MUCH TO EAT

A medium orange weighs 6oz. Aim to eat at least one citrus fruit daily. Eat as a snack, in salads, and in cooking. Also make use of the rind. A 6oz. glass of orange juice is a "portion" of fruit but lacks the fiber content.

KEY BENEFITS

The flavanone hesperidin is an important phyto-chemical in oranges. Flavanones are found mainly in citrus fruit and protect the body from free radical damage with their antioxidant actions.

● **CHOLESTEROL LEVELS**
Oranges (like apples) are a good source of pectin, a soluble fiber with modest effects on lowering choles-terol. Flavanones may also lower cholesterol levels.

● **BREAST CANCER**
In animal studies, drinking double-strength orange juice inhibited the growth of breast cancer cells. Hesperidin was identified

as an anticancer agent, but is believed to work with other phyto-chemicals in orange juice.

● **SUPPORTS VITAMIN C**
Flavanones promote the absorption and activity of vitamin C, which helps make collagen for healthy skin, defend the body against bacteria, and keep blood vessels healthy.

ORANGE: OTHER PHYTOCHEMICALS

OTHER FLAVONOIDS	pp.34–35
PHENOLIC ACIDS	pp.56–57
LIMONENE	pp.102

NUTRITIONAL VALUES
Quantities per 4oz.

CALORIES	37
FIBER	1.7g
VITAMIN C	54mg

GRAPEFRUIT

May protect against stomach cancer

Can benefit lung function ◆ Good source of vitamin C

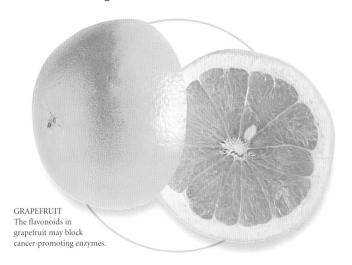

GRAPEFRUIT
The flavonoids in
grapefruit may block
cancer-promoting enzymes.

MAXIMIZING THE BENEFITS

Naringenin is well absorbed by the body. Eat the membranes and pith for maximum effect. Grapefruit is at its best when fresh and chilled as the vitamin C content is maximized.

HOW MUCH TO EAT

Half a grapefruit weighs 3½oz, and although low in calories, it does not have any special fat-burning powers. Note: grapefruit juice should not be drunk with certain drugs, e.g., antihistamines, as it can change their action in the body.

KEY BENEFITS

Grapefruit is a source of the flavanone naringenin, which gives a distinct bitter taste. It is an anti-oxidant and has choles-terol-lowering properties. Flavanones also have antibacterial action.

● **WHEEZE**
Eating vitamin C-rich fruit can benefit lung function. Italian children who ate citrus fruit or kiwifruit on most days in winter had fewer wheezing problems than those who ate them less than once a week.

● **LUNG AND STOMACH CANCER**
Numerous studies have shown citrus fruit to have a protective effect against cancer, especially stomach cancer. Flavanones may help, as may vitamin C, which blocks the forma-tion of nitrates (p.109) into potentially carcinogenic nitrosamines. A Hawaiian study found that regular grapefruit eaters had a 50 percent lower risk of developing lung cancer.

GRAPEFRUIT: OTHER PHYTOCHEMICALS

OTHER FLAVONOIDS	pp.34–35
PHENOLIC ACIDS	pp.56–57
LIMONOIDS	p.102

NUTRITIONAL VALUES
Quantities per 4oz.

CALORIES	20
FIBER	0.9g
VITAMIN C	24mg
FOLATE	18mcg

GUIDE TO PHYTOESTROGENS

The differences between traditional Asian and Western diets and the lower incidence of certain diseases by Asian communities is being studied closely by researchers in search of a clue to the effects of diet and lifestyle.

Population studies show that people living in East Asian countries, such as China and Japan, who enjoy a traditional diet have a much lower risk of heart disease, breast and prostate cancer, hip fracture (from osteoporosis), and menopausal symptoms compared to people in the West. Research also indicates that the increased incidence of risk is probably due to diet and lifestyle changes rather than genetic differences.

PHYTOESTROGENS

One key factor differentiating traditional Asian diets from Western diets is that they have a much higher intake of phytochemicals known as phytoestrogens. Phytoestrogens are a type of "plant estrogen" and have a similar structure to the female sex hormone, estrogen. Their action in the body is far weaker than the true hormone, yet they have been shown to have biological effects in women, such as increasing the length of the menstrual cycle, for example.

Phytoestrogens have the ability to act as estrogens or anti-estrogens, that is, they can either mimic or reduce the action of natural estrogen in specific parts of the body. For this reason they are thought to help balance estrogen levels over a lifetime. Phytoestrogen-rich foods also offer health benefits that are separate from these hormonal effects.

There are three main types of phytoestrogens: isoflavones (a type of flavonoid, see p.34), coumestrol, and lignans. Resveratrol (pp.68–69), a type of stilbene, also belongs to the phytoestrogen family. All are phenolic compounds, and the best food sources include soy beans, lentils, garbanzo beans, legumes, bean sprouts, linseeds, and wholegrains, with much smaller amounts found in fruit and vegetables.

ISOFLAVONES

There are four main types of isoflavones: genistein, daidzein, formononetin, and biochanin. To be well absorbed by the body, they must be further broken down by bacteria in the colon (large intestine). Recent studies show that following a plant food-rich, high carbohydrate, lower-fat diet actually encourages more of these isoflavones to be absorbed –

no doubt because such a diet helps promote a good balance of bacteria in the bowel *(see p.21)*. More evidence for the role of bacteria is that antibiotic treatment, which kills off bacteria, can block the proper absorption of phytoestrogens.

Isoflavones are the most studied phytoestrogens – especially those found in soy beans, which are a key source of phytoestrogens in Eastern diets. It is estimated that people living in Japan and China currently consume 20-50mg isoflavones a day compared to less than 1mg by people living in the West. Researchers suggest that the lower risk of breast cancer and prostate cancer in Asia may be due to a lifetime exposure to isoflavone-rich foods.

HEALTH BENEFITS

The effects of phytoestrogens in the body have been more thoroughly researched than most other phyto-chemicals. Even so, there is still uncertainty about what impact they really have on our health. Numerous studies have linked eating foods rich in phytoestrogens, especially iso-flavone-rich soy, with potentially positive health benefits relating to heart disease and, to a lesser extent, cancers, bone strength, and post-menopausal health. These effects may be due to phytoestrogens, but other nutrients and phytochemicals in foods could also be offering benefit. For example, soy beans are a good source of protein, fiber, omega-3 fats, potassium, folate, and a range of phytochemicals such as phyto-sterols *(p.97)* and saponins *(p.103)*.

Isoflavones have antioxidant abilities, too, and the protein in soy is also necessary for its cholesterol-lowering effect *(see p.50)*. Eating a variety of plant-based foods and foods rich in phytoestrogens may be the best way forward.

Eating too many phytoestrogens may have negative effects on health *(p.110)*, and healthy limits for phyto-estrogen intakes for all age groups are currently being researched. The amounts recommended for specific health benefits, for example, for lowering cholesterol *(see p.50)*, are considered "safe." Caution is advised with concentrated isoflavone supplements (unless taken on medical advice) or large amounts of fortified foods *(p.26)*. Listed below are the main food sources of phytoestrogens:

◆ **ISOFLAVONES**

Soy beans, tofu, soy milk, soy yogurt and cheese, roasted soy nuts, miso, soy flour (in many processed foods), soy flakes, garbanzo beans, lentils, gram, pinto beans, haricot beans, peanuts, milo.

◆ **COUMESTROL**

Mung bean sprouts, alfalfa sprouts, soy bean sprouts.

◆ **LIGNANS**

Linseeds, wholewheat, rye, barley, sesame seeds, pumpkin seeds, sunflower seeds, legumes, cranberries, apples, pears, carrots, cherries, onion, corn, broccoli (and found to some extent in most grain, fruit, and vegetables).

SOY BEANS

Helps lower cholesterol levels

Good for general heart health • May benefit bones

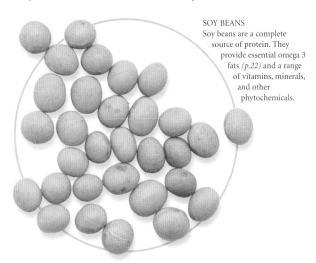

SOY BEANS
Soy beans are a complete
source of protein. They
provide essential omega 3
fats (p.22) and a range
of vitamins, minerals,
and other
phytochemicals.

MAXIMIZING THE BENEFITS

Isoflavones are not reduced by normal cooking processes, and are best absorbed by people who eat a healthy high-carbo-hydrate, lower-fat diet. Soy beans also contain omega 3 fats and are an excellent source of protein.

HOW MUCH TO EAT

3½oz. cooked soy beans provides about ½oz. soy protein and 40mg isoflavones. One serving of soy foods daily may provide East Asian levels of isoflavones. Use in soups and casseroles.

KEY BENEFITS

Soy beans are the best source of the isoflavone phytochemicals genistein and daidzein (p.48).

● LOWERS CHOLESTEROL
Eating a diet containing 1oz. soy protein each day can lower cholesterol levels by up to 10 percent. Eating less will reduce cholesterol by smaller amounts. In the U.S., foods that have at least ¼oz. soy protein (and include isoflavones) per serving can carry a health claim to this effect.

● HEART DISEASE
Isoflavone-rich soy foods have been shown to have beneficial actions that may protect against the oxidation of "bad" LDL cholesterol, reduce the risk of blood clots, and help keep blood vessels flexible (so reducing risk of athersclerosis).

● BONE HEALTH
Compared to animal protein, soy protein reduces the amount of calcium (needed for bones) lost in the urine.

SOY BEAN: OTHER PHYTOCHEMICALS

PROTEASE INHIBITORS	pp.94–95
PHYTIC ACID	p.96
SAPONINS	p.103

NUTRITIONAL VALUES
Quantities per 4oz., cooked

CALORIES	140
FIBER	6.1g
POTASSIUM	510mg

TOFU & SOY MILK

Has anticancer effects ◆ Linked to lower risk of

prostate cancer ◆ Source of calcium and omega 3 fats

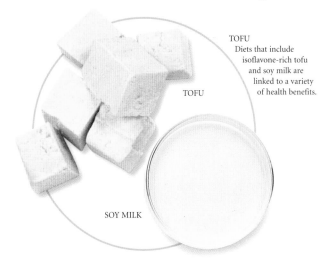

TOFU
Diets that include
isoflavone-rich tofu
and soy milk are
linked to a variety
of health benefits.

TOFU

TOFU

SOY MILK

MAXIMIZING INTAKE

Isoflavone content is preserved when tofu and soy milk are made from soy beans and will survive cooking; choose calcium-fortified brands, especially if using soy milk in place of dairy products.

HOW MUCH TO EAT

Typical servings of tofu are 3–4oz., and soy milk 6–8oz. These provide around ⅓–½oz. protein and 20-25mg isoflavones (the content varies between brands). Use soy milk as you would cow's milk, and include tofu in stir fries, rice dishes, and kabobs.

KEY BENEFITS

Isoflavones are the key phytochemicals found in tofu and soy milk, made from isoflavone-rich soy beans. Studies suggest that isoflavones may help fight cancer in several ways: by their anti-estrogen effects; by blocking the enzymes needed for cancer cell growth; by restricting the blood supply to cancer cells; and inhibiting any free radical damage.

● **BREAST CANCER**
Japanese women have a low risk of developing breast cancer and have high levels of isoflavones in their blood compared to Western women. Their lifetime exposure to

isoflavones may influence the body to adapt, lowering the risk of breast cancer.

● **PROSTRATE CANCER**
A 20-year study of men in the U.S. found that those who drank soy milk more than once a day had a 70 percent reduced risk of developing cancer compared to those who didn't.

TOFU/SOY: OTHER PHYTOCHEMICALS

PROTEASE INHIBITORS	p.94
PHYTIC ACID	pp.95–96
PHYTOSTEROLS	p.97

NUTRITIONAL VALUES
Soy milk per 4oz.

CALORIES	36
FIBER	1.2g
CALCIUM	120mg
VITAMIN E	1.5mg

LENTILS

May help manage menopausal symptoms and maintain

bone strength ◆ Source of protein and iron

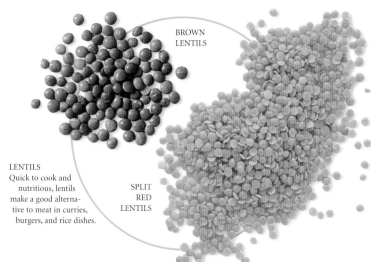

BROWN
LENTILS

LENTILS
Quick to cook and
nutritious, lentils
make a good alterna-
tive to meat in curries,
burgers, and rice dishes.

SPLIT
RED
LENTILS

MAXIMIZING THE BENEFITS

While soy foods are the richest sources of genistein and daidzein isoflavones, garbanzo beans and lentils contain a good balance of other isoflavones. Mixing these foods is an ideal way to opti-mize isoflavones and increase lignan intake.

HOW MUCH TO EAT

An average serving of cooked lentils is 4¼oz (3tbsp). Menopausal women could include foods rich in phyto-estrogens daily for at least 12 weeks as part of a healthy lifestyle to see if symptoms lessen.

KEY BENEFITS

Lentils contain a very small amount of isoflavones, and are quite a good source of lignan phytoestrogens.

● MENOPAUSAL SYMPTOMS

Asian women who regu-larly eat isoflavone-rich foods suffer few menopausal problems. Some studies suggest that eating isoflavone-rich diets can improve menopausal symptoms, while others show limited or no benefit.

● BONE HEALTH

The hormone estrogen helps to maintain bone strength, and the risk of osteoporosis (brittle

bones) increases greatly at menopause as estrogen levels decline. Studies suggest that isoflavones may help prevent bones from weakening, but more research is needed before recommendations can be made. A lifelong balanced diet and active lifestyle is also essential for bone health.

LENTILS: OTHER PHYTOCHEMICALS

PHENOLIC ACIDS pp.56–57	
CONDENSED TANNINS p.67	
PHYTIC ACID pp.95–96	

NUTRITIONAL VALUES
Quantities per 4oz., boiled

CALORIES	104
FIBER	3.8g
IRON	3.5mg
FOLATE	30mcg

BEAN SPROUTS

Traditional remedy for arthritis and menopausal

symptoms ◆ May benefit cholesterol levels

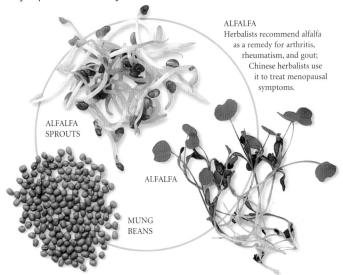

ALFALFA
Herbalists recommend alfalfa
as a remedy for arthritis,
rheumatism, and gout;
Chinese herbalists use
it to treat menopausal
symptoms.

ALFALFA
SPROUTS

ALFALFA

MUNG
BEANS

MAXIMIZING THE BENEFITS

Fresh sprouts can be grown at home in 2-3 days. Soak dry mung beans or alfalfa seeds overnight, drain, store in a dark place, and rinse daily until the seeds or beans have begun to sprout.

HOW MUCH TO EAT

An average serving of mung beans is 1½oz. (2tbsp). Use bean sprouts soon after purchase: rinse well and add to sandwiches, salads, garnishes, and stir fries. Soy sprouts must be cooked before being eaten.

KEY BENEFITS

Coumestrol is a phyto-chemical found almost exclusively in alfalfa, soy-bean, and mung sprouts. It is a potent phytoestrogen, and laboratory studies reveal antioxidant and anti-inflammatory abilities. Coumestrol intakes in Western diets are very low compared to East Asian diets, which regularly include bean sprouts.

● **PROSTRATE CANCER**
An American study com-pared the diets of 83 men with prostate cancer to the diets of 107 cancer-free "controls." The controls ate more foods containing coumestrol and isoflavones, and the

overall results suggested a protective link between prostate cancer risk and these phytoestrogens.

● **ALFALFA**
Alfalfa has cholesterol-lowering abilities, which are largely due to phyto-chemicals called saponins (p.103). People with lupus may be allergic to alfalfa and other bean sprouts.

ALFALFA SPROUTS: OTHER PHYTOCHEMICALS

PHENOLIC ACIDS pp.56–57	
SAPONINS p.103	

NUTRITIONAL VALUES
Quantities per 4oz.

CALORIES	24
FIBER	1.7g
FOLATE	36mcg

WHOLEWHEAT

Helps reduce the risk of heart disease

Promotes bowel health ◆ Good source of fiber

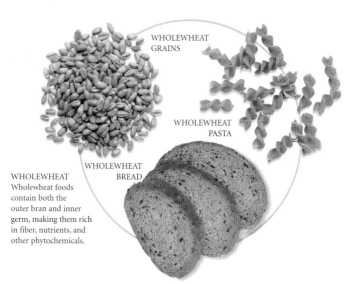

WHOLEWHEAT
GRAINS

WHOLEWHEAT
PASTA

WHOLEWHEAT
BREAD

WHOLEWHEAT
Wholewheat foods
contain both the
outer bran and inner
germ, making them rich
in fiber, nutrients, and
other phytochemicals.

MAXIMIZING THE BENEFITS

Lignan is found in the outer layer of wheat grains, so eat whole-wheat rather than refined wheat foods for maximum lignan intake. Wheat intol-erance can be over-diagnosed and is best assessed by a doctor or registered dietitian.

HOW MUCH TO EAT

One slice of whole-wheat bread weighing 1¼oz is equivalent to one serving. Three daily servings of any wholegrain food may help reduce the risk of cancer and heart disease by up to 30%.

KEY BENEFITS

Wholewheat foods are a source of lignans – phyto-chemicals that are wide-spread in vegetables and cereals. Lignans are broken down by bacteria in the gut to form enterolactone and enterodiol lignans, which exert biological effects in the body. Diets rich in wholewheat help protect against heart disease and cancers.

● **HEART DISEASE**
A Finnish study found that middle-aged men with high blood levels of enterolactone had a 65 percent lower risk of having a heart attack than men with low levels. In laboratory studies lignans

can act as antioxidants and inhibit "bad" LDL cholesterol oxidation.

● **BOWEL HEALTH**
Wholewheat is a good source of fiber, fructo-oligosaccharides (p.98), and resistant starch, maintaining healthy levels of gut flora and keeping the bowel regular.

WHOLEWHEAT: OTHER PHYTOCHEMICALS

PROTEASE INHIBITORS	p.94
PHYTIC ACID	pp.95–96
PHYTOSTEROLS	p.97

NUTRITIONAL VALUES
Quantities per 4oz., bread

CALORIES	215
FIBER	5.8g
IRON	2.7mg
POTASSIUM	230mg

LINSEEDS

Has anticancer effects ◆ May help manage
menopausal symptoms ◆ Source of fiber and omega-3 fats

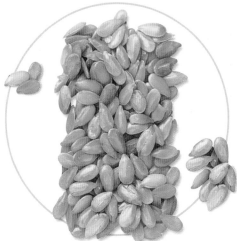

LINSEEDS
Linseeds are rich
in heart-healthy
omega-3 fats
(p.22) and may
help to lower
cholesterol levels.

MAXIMIZING THE BENEFITS

Bacteria in the intestine must first break down lignans before they can be absorbed. A plant-food rich, high carbohydrate, lower-fat diet helps keep up healthy levels of gut bacteria to maximize lignan absorption. Choose precracked organic golden linseeds and store in the refrigerator.

HOW MUCH TO EAT

1tbsp. will meet omega-3 fat requirements and keep the bowel regular. Sprinkle on cereal or salads, stir into yogurt, and add to home-baked goods.

KEY BENEFITS

Linseeds are the richest food source of the phytochemicals known as lignans. Of the 100 or so different types of lignans, only two are known to act as phytoestrogens. Lignans are also antioxidants, which protect against free radical cell damage. Linseeds can also help to keep the bowel healthy.

● CANCER

Population studies link high blood levels of enterolactone *(see p.54)* with a lower risk of breast and colon cancer. Lignans also show anticancer effects in animal and laboratory studies.

● WOMEN'S HEALTH

Studies suggest that soy and linseed in the diets of menopausal women may help to alleviate menopausal symptoms. Other studies show no clear benefit, and research continues. Linseeds are also rich in omega 3-fats, which may improve inflammatory conditions.

LINSEED: OTHER PHYTOCHEMICALS

| PHYTOSTEROLS p.97 |
| PHENOLIC ACIDS pp.56–57 |
| PHYTIC ACID pp.95–96 |

NUTRITIONAL VALUES
Quantities per 4oz.

CALORIES	396
FIBER	37g
OMEGA-3 FATS	22g
MAGNESIUM	350mg

GUIDE TO OTHER PHENOLIC COMPOUNDS

In addition to flavonoids, another 4,000 different phenolic compounds have so far been identified. They range from simple phenolic acids to more complex condensed tannins and can be divided into about ten classes.

Foods rich in phenolics generally contain flavonoids, too, so population studies that show a link between high intakes of flavonoids and a reduced risk of heart disease and stroke typically hold true for other phenolics. In addition, laboratory and population studies point toward cancer protection from many phenolic-rich foods.

The interest in phenolic compounds initially stemmed from how they could be used in the classification of plants, and for their effects on nutrient absorption. Phenolics can bind with minerals such as iron and zinc in the intestine and reduce their absorption. Vitamin C-rich foods (p.23), and possibly foods rich in betacarotene (pp.76–77) help to counteract this effect – yet another example of the importance of a varied diet for good health.

USES OF PHENOLIC COMPOUNDS

Phenolic compounds are widely utilized in the food industry as natural preservatives, for example, or to clarify or clean wines and beer. Other industrial applications include the production of paper, ink, paint, rubber, and also as leather tanning agents. A tannin can be defined as a compound that can transform animal hides into leather due to its ability to form stable complexes with the protein in animal hide. Tannins used for industrial purposes are usually derived from the bark of oak trees or from tree galls.

There are two main tannins in plants: hydrolyzable tannins, such as those found in walnuts and other nuts; and condensed tannins, found, for example, in dark-colored legumes and grapes. It is these tannins that give distinctive astringency to food and drinks such as wine – caused by a mild reaction between the tannins and the proteins in the saliva of the mouth.

Today, phenolic compounds are intriguing scientists and dietitians alike with the possible health benefits they bring. They exhibit antioxidant, anticancer, anti-inflammatory, antibacterial, antithrombotic and blood vessel relaxing effects (probably via increased release of nitric oxide).

Laboratory studies may suggest certain health benefits, but more human intervention studies *(p.29)* are needed before any conclusions can be made about their direct health effects once inside the body.

However, the research conducted so far suggests that phenolic compounds appear to be reasonably well absorbed and do play some role in helping to protect against heart disease, stoke, cancer, bacterial infections, circulation problems, and the general effects of aging.

SOURCES OF PHENOLIC COMPOUNDS

Phenolics are widespread in fruit, vegetables, herbs, wholegrains, seeds, and nuts but some foods are particularly rich in these compounds. Examples of these foods include hot chilis, pungent turmeric, rich red wine, tangy cranberries, plump blueberries, sensual strawberries, and comforting potatoes. Phenolics are not usually destroyed by cooking, but they are generally attracted to water, meaning that they will leach into the water they are cooked in. In order to optimize intakes, keep cooking times short and/or consume cooking water, for example, the juice from stewed plums or pears.

Use the following guide to key sources of phenolic compounds *(right)*, together with the following pages of phytochemical and food profiles, in order to maximize your intakes of these compounds and enjoy the tastes, textures, and colors of phenolic-rich foods.

PHENOLIC ACIDS:

◆ **HYDROXYBENZOIC ACIDS, E.G., GALLIC ACID, ELLAGIC ACID, SALICYLIC ACID (SALICYLATE)**
Raspberries, strawberries, blackberries, walnuts, pecans, grapes, tea, cranberries.
Note: most dried herbs and spices are rich in salicylate.

◆ **HYDROXYCINNAMIC ACIDS E.G., FERULIC ACID, CAFFEIC ACID, COUMARIC ACID, CURCUMIN, CHLOROGENIC ACID**
Blueberries, pears, apples, oranges, lettuce, potatoes, grapefruit, coffee beans, cherries, endive, sunflower seeds, turmeric, ginger, herbs such as rosemary, sage, marjoram, thyme.

OTHER PHENOLIC COMPOUNDS:

◆ **CAPSAICIN**
Chilis, peppers.

◆ **CONDENSED TANNINS (PROANTHOCYANIDINS)**
Cranberries, lentils, black-eyed peas, black gram, red kidney beans, red wine, grapes (dark and light), grape seeds, pears, apples, chocolate.

◆ **A STILBENE, RESVERATROL**
Grape skin, red wine, peanuts, mulberries.

◆ **COUMARINS**
Citrus fruits, cassava, parsley, celeriac, celery, parsnips, carrots, cilantro, fennel, figs.

STRAWBERRY

Has anticancer effects

Raises body antioxidant levels ◆ Rich source of vitamin C

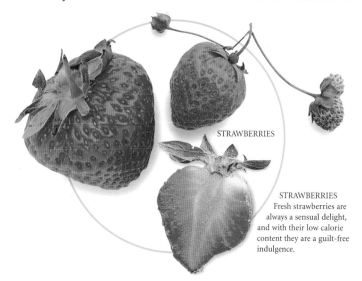

STRAWBERRIES

STRAWBERRIES
Fresh strawberries are
always a sensual delight,
and with their low calorie
content they are a guilt-free
indulgence.

MAXIMIZING THE BENEFITS

The fresher they are, the higher the antioxidant value of strawberries. Their vitamin C and folate content is particularly vunerable, so store them in the fridge and and eat soon after purchase. Like all berries, they are a good source of salicylic acid.

HOW MUCH TO EAT

Eight strawberries weigh about 3oz.; 20 strawberries (8oz.) has proven effects on antioxidant levels in the blood. Eat as a snack, in fruit salads, and with cold meats and cheese.

KEY BENEFITS

Strawberries are a key source of ellagic acid, a phenolic acid that has potent anticarcinogenic activity and also acts as an antioxidant.

● CANCER

Numerous laboratory studies indicate that ellagic acid can inhibit the growth of tumors, for example, of the tongue, oesophagus, and the lungs. It may do this by blocking the action of carcinogens or by reducing the absorption of carcinogens from the intestine. Eating strawberries regularly as part of a healthy diet has also been linked to reduced risk of prostate cancer.

● ANTIOXIDANT ACTIVITY

Strawberries rank high on the fresh fruit and vegetables antioxidant scale (p.23). In a study of elderly women, 8oz. or 20 strawberries eaten daily significantly increased their antioxidant blood activity, showing that the antioxidants in strawberries (for example, ellagic acid and vitamin C) can be used by the body.

STRAWBERRY: OTHER PHYTOCHEMICALS

FLAVONOIDS pp.34–35

NUTRITIONAL VALUES
Quantities per 40z.

CALORIES	27
FIBER	1.1g
VITAMIN C	77mg
FOLATE	20mcg

WALNUT

Helps protect against heart disease

Lowers cholesterol levels ◆ Good source of omega-3 fats

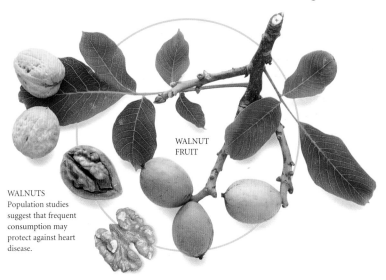

WALNUT
FRUIT

WALNUTS
Population studies
suggest that frequent
consumption may
protect against heart
disease.

MAXIMIZING THE BENEFITS

Crack fresh walnuts from the shell, or buy vacuum packed. Store walnuts in an airtight container in the refrigerator, and use soon after purchase. Chopped walnuts become rancid quickly.

HOW MUCH TO EAT

Four walnuts (1oz.) will provide a healthy amount of essential omega-3 fats. Walnuts add rich bite to snacks, salads, greens, rice, fish, or chicken dishes and desserts. Walnut oil also adds flavor – and omega-3 fats – to dishes.

KEY BENEFITS

Walnuts are a source of the phytochemical ellagic acid. They have an astringent taste due to their ellagic acid-based tannin content.

● **HEART DISEASE**
Walnuts have a number of attributes that may help to protect against heart disease: antioxidants such as ellagic acid, selenium and vitamin E; and also a heart-healthy balance between omega-3 fats *(p.22)* and polyun-saturated fats.

● **CHOLESTEROL LEVELS**
Trials show that incorporating walnuts into the typical Mediterranean or

Japanese diet can lead to additional decreases in "bad" LDL cholesterol. Subjects ate an average of 2oz. walnuts a day in place of other sources of fat so the total fat and calorie content was similar for the test diet and the typical diet.

WALNUT: OTHER PHYTOCHEMICALS

| FLAVONOIDS pp.34–35 |
| PHYTOSTEROLS p.97 |
| BIOGENIC AMINES p.104 |

NUTRITIONAL VALUES
Quantities per 4oz.

CALORIES	688
FIBRE	3.5g
OMEGA-3 FATS	7.5g
POTASSIUM	450mg
VITAMIN E	3.9mg
SELENIUM	8mcg

PECAN

Has anticancer effects ◆ Lowers cholesterol levels

Source of potassium and selenium

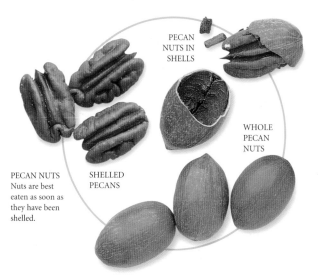

PECAN
NUTS IN
SHELLS

WHOLE
PECAN
NUTS

PECAN NUTS
Nuts are best
eaten as soon as
they have been
shelled.

SHELLED
PECANS

MAXIMIZING THE BENEFITS

Being high in polyunsaturated fat, pecans are best eaten fresh from the shell or if preshelled, stored in an airtight container in a cool place.

HOW MUCH TO EAT

Five pecans weigh 1oz. Eating this amount of any type of nut at least five times a week is associated with a 30-50% lower risk of heart disease. Nuts are recommended as a regular part of the American DASH (Dietary Approaches to Stop Hypertension) diet for high blood pressure.

KEY BENEFITS

The pecan nut is another important source of ellagic acid, and it also includes good amounts of vital vitamin E, selenium, magnesium, potassium, and polyunsaturated fats.

● CANCER

Laboratory studies with cancer cells show that ellagic acid not only blocks the action of carcinogens, it can trigger "apoptosis" – when the cancer cell is essentially forced to commit suicide.

● CHOLESTEROL LEVELS

Test subjects ate 2½oz. of pecans daily for eight weeks as part of a varied, self-selected diet.

Cholesterol levels in test subjects were modestly lowered compared to those test subjects who did not eat pecans. Note: weight gain is a potential problem over time if foods are added, rather than substituted, in the diet.

PECAN: OTHER PHYTOCHEMICALS

FLAVONOIDS	pp.34–35
BIOGENIC AMINES	p.104
PHYTOSTEROLS	p.97

NUTRITIONAL VALUES
Quantities per 4oz.

CALORIES	689
FIBER	4.6g
POTASSIUM	520mg
MAGNESIUM	130mg
VITAMIN E	4.3mg
SELENIUM	12mcg

BLACKBERRY

Has anticancer effects ◆ Good low-fat source of
vitamin E ◆ May trigger reactions in sensitive people

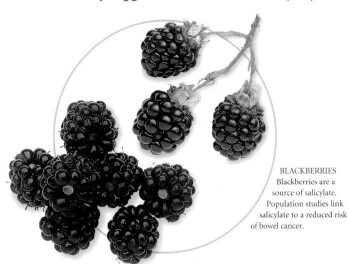

BLACKBERRIES
Blackberries are a
source of salicylate.
Population studies link
salicylate to a reduced risk
of bowel cancer.

MAXIMIZING THE BENEFITS

Fresh blackberries contain the highest quantities of phenolic acids, vitamin C, and folate. Cooked black-berries contain as much vitamin E and fiber. Other berries, dried fruit spices, and herbs are salicylate sources, and smaller amounts are found in most fruit and vege-tables. Some people are salicylate-sensitive *(see p.110).*

HOW MUCH TO EAT

Fifteen blackberries weigh 3oz. Eat as a nutritious dessert or snack, or bake or juice.

KEY BENEFITS

Blackberries are a good source of salicylate, a hydroxybenzoic phenolic acid that plants produce to fight infection. The anti-inflammatory, pain-killing drug aspirin is produced from salicylate, which was originally ex-tracted from willow trees.

● **BOWEL CANCER**
Laboratory studies show that salicylate can inhibit the development of colon (large bowel) cancer cells. The effect of supplemen-tary salicylate on bowel cancer is being studied, too.

● **HEART DISEASE**
American researchers have suggested that

dietary salicylate may reduce the risk of heart disease. However, current intakes are not likely to be high enough to benefit bowel or heart health as modern farming methods aim to minimize plant infection, and therefore plants produce less protective salicylate.

BLACKBERRY: OTHER PHYTOCHEMICALS

FLAVONOIDS pp.34–35	
OTHER PHENOLIC ACIDS pp.56–57	
LIGNANS pp.54–55	

NUTRITIONAL VALUES
Quantities per 4oz.

CALORIES	25
FIBER	3.1g
FOLATE	34mg
VITAMIN E	2.4mg

BLUEBERRY

Supports strength of small blood vessels ◆ May delay the
effects of aging ◆ Very high antioxidant ability

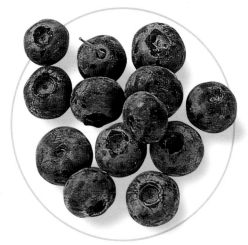

BLUEBERRIES
Blueberries and
bilberries make a
tasty fresh dessert
and are popular
in muffins and
pancakes.

MAXIMIZING THE BENEFITS

Eating the equivalent
of half a cup of blue-
berries has been bene-
ficial in animal studies.
A recent human study
showed no significant
increase in blood
antioxidant capacity
after drinking 2 cups
blueberry juice. More
research is needed to
clarify how blueberry
components exert their
benefits in the body.

HOW MUCH TO EAT

A potentially beneficial
serving of blueberries
is 2½oz. (about 30
berries). Blueberries
taste good in baked
goods and freeze well.

KEY BENEFITS

Blueberries, and the European equivalent bilberries,
are rich in phenolic acid
and flavonoid phyto-
chemicals, and have the
highest antioxidant ability
of all fresh fruit. Blue-
berries also have effective
anti-inflammatory, anti–
blood clotting, and anti-
bacterial effects *(see
Cranberries, p.67)*.

● **PROTECTS
BLOOD VESSELS**
The anti-inflammatory
action of blueberries
helps control the integrity
of capillaries (small blood
vessels) by stopping free
radical damage from
making them leaky. Re-
searchers suggest this

effect might help protect
against the capillary
damage associated with
diabetes, which can lead to
eye and kidney problems.

● **ANTI-AGING**
Older rats who ate the
equivalent of half a cup of
blueberries daily for eight
weeks showed an improve-
ment in age-related decline
in short-term memory
and coordination.

BLUEBERRY: OTHER PHYTOCHEMICALS

FLAVONOIDS	pp.34–35
CONDENSED TANNINS	p.67

NUTRITIONAL VALUES
Quantities per 4oz.

CALORIES	56
FIBER	2.7g
VITAMIN C	13mg

PEAR

Antibacterial action ◆ Has anticancer effects

Useful for allergy diets

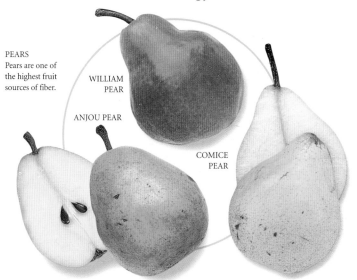

PEARS
Pears are one of
the highest fruit
sources of fiber.

WILLIAM
PEAR

ANJOU PEAR

COMICE
PEAR

MAXIMIZING THE BENEFITS

Chlorogenic acid, one of the hydroxy-cinnamic acids in pears, tends to accumulate in pear skin, so wash well and eat whole whether fresh or cooked. This helps to maximize its fiber content, too.

HOW MUCH TO EAT

A medium pear weighs 4–5oz. Fresh pears make a convenient, energy-boosting snack, or use in fruit salads or bake or stew. Peeled, stewed, and puréed pears with no added sugar make an ideal first weaning food.

KEY BENEFITS

Pears are a source of hydroxycinnamic acids, which act as good anti-oxidants and may block the formation of cancer-causing agents. Hydroxy-cinnamic acids can be absorbed by the body.

● ANTIBACTERIAL

Laboratory studies show that hydroxycinnamic acids can inhibit the growth of potentially harmful bacteria such as Shigella sonnei, a cause of severe gastroenteritis.

● CANCER

Hydroxycinnamic acids may help to protect against colon cancer, possibly by binding

nitrates in the stomach and blocking their conversion to potentially carcinogenic compounds called nitrosamines (p.109).

● FOOD ALLERGY

Pears are one of the least likely foods to trigger an allergic reaction and so are used as part of an exclusion diet to investigate food intolerance.

PEAR: OTHER PHYTOCHEMICALS

| FLAVONOIDS pp.34–35 |
| CONDENSED TANNINS p.67 |

NUTRITIONAL VALUES
Quantities per 4oz.

CALORIES	40
FIBER	2.2g
POTASSIUM	150mg
VITAMIN C	6mg

PLUM & PRUNE

Have anticancer effects ◆ Very high

antioxidant ability ◆ Source of iron and potassium

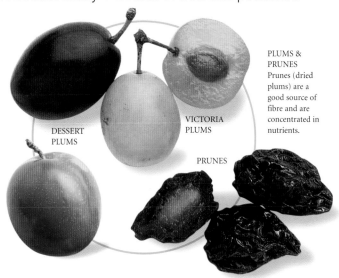

PLUMS & PRUNES
Prunes (dried plums) are a good source of fibre and are concentrated in nutrients.

VICTORIA PLUMS

DESSERT PLUMS

PRUNES

MAXIMIZING THE BENEFITS

Fresh or dried plums offer potential antioxidant benefits. Stewing won't destroy hydroxycinnamic acids, although some will leach into the cooking water. Prunes are useful for low-fat baking: simply replace half the fat in a cake recipe with puréed prune.

HOW MUCH TO EAT

Three small plums (3oz.) or three prunes are equivalent to a portion of fruit. Eat fresh plums as a snack or on cereal, or bake or stew. Prunes also make a good snack.

KEY BENEFITS

Plums and prunes (the dried version of plums) are a source of a hydroxy-cinnamic acid called ferulic acid, and other phenolic phytochemicals, making them a rich source of antioxidants.

● BOWEL HEALTH
Hydroxycinnamic acids such as ferulic acid have been associated with a reduced risk of colon cancer. One way they might offer protection is by inhibiting formation of the potent cell-damaging free radical, peroxynitrite, found in the colon. Prunes are known for their laxative effect; this may be due to the sugars they contain.

● ANTIOXIDANT ABILITY
Because prunes are dried, they rank very highly on the ORAC antioxidant scale *(see p.25)*. This means they may offer a high level of defense against damaging free radicals. Compared to fresh plums, they are also more concentrated in nutrients, especially iron and potassium.

PLUM: OTHER PHYTOCHEMICALS

FLAVONOIDS	pp.34–35
CONDENSED TANNINS	p.67
CAROTENOIDS	pp.72–73

NUTRITIONAL VALUES
Quantities per 4oz., plums

CALORIES	36
FIBER	1.6g
POTASSIUM	240mg

POTATO

Rich in healthy energy ◆ Useful source of
vitamin C and iron ◆ Green or sprouted potatoes are toxic

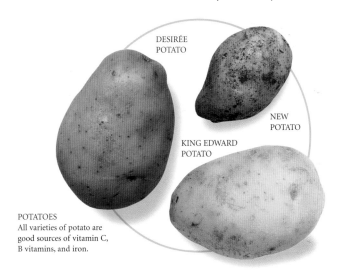

DESIRÉE
POTATO

NEW
POTATO

KING EDWARD
POTATO

POTATOES
All varieties of potato are
good sources of vitamin C,
B vitamins, and iron.

MAXIMIZING THE BENEFITS

Scrubbed thoroughly before cooking, new or baked potatoes are a good choice since their vitamin C and hydroxycinnamic acids tend to concentrate just under the skin. Cold boiled potatoes are a good source of resistant starch that helps promote healthy gut bacteria (p.21).

HOW MUCH TO EAT

An average serving of boiled potatoes or a baked potato is 6oz. Bake, boil, mash, or roast in a little oil to keep added fat low.

KEY BENEFITS

The humble potato is a source of hydroxy-cinnamic acids, giving it antioxidant abilities. It is also a surprisingly good source of vitamin C, B vitamins, and iron, due to the relatively large portions eaten. Avoid sprouted or green potatoes, which are high in a toxic phyto-chemical (see p.111).

● **WEIGHT CONTROL**
Potatoes have a bad name for being fattening, but they are actually a filling, low-fat source of nutrients and polyphenols, and should not be avoided by the weight conscious – unless always deep fried! They do have a high glycemic index (GI, p.21), meaning they can raise blood sugar levels quickly. Serving potatoes with lower GI foods – for example, peas, beans, or topped with natural yogurt – will lower the GI of the meal and make it more satisfying.

POTATO: OTHER PHYTOCHEMICALS

FLAVONOIDS	pp.34–35
GLYCOALKALOIDS	p.111
OTHER PHENOLIC ACIDS	pp.56–57

NUTRITIONAL VALUES
Quantities per 4oz., boiled

CALORIES	66
FIBER	1.5g
POTASSIUM	430mg
VITAMIN C	15mg
IRON	1.6mg

TURMERIC

Has anticancer effects ◆ Digestion stimulant
Anti-inflammatory agent

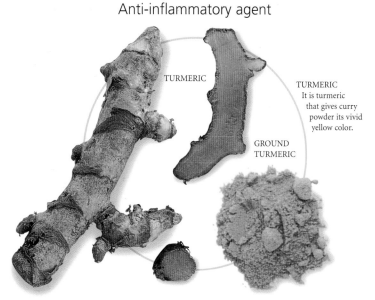

TURMERIC

TURMERIC
It is turmeric
that gives curry
powder its vivid
yellow color.

GROUND
TURMERIC

MAXIMIZING THE BENEFITS

Turmeric is a member of the ginger family, and while sometimes used fresh in Asian cooking, the dried, powdered form of the root is commonly used worldwide.

HOW MUCH TO EAT

One small teaspoon of curcumin weighs ⅒oz. but since it is a dried, concentrated spice, only small amounts are needed in cooking. Use turmeric to add warm color and flavor to rice and potato dishes, as well as curries and pickles.

KEY BENEFITS

Turmeric is the most important source of the phytochemical curcumin (a type of hydroxy-cinnamic acid). Turmeric is being investigated for its anticancer and anti-inflammatory effects.

● BOWEL CANCER
British cancer specialists are testing oral curcumin-rich capsules on people with colon cancer after identifying that this cancer is much lower in Asian communities, where turmeric is used frequently.

● DIGESTIVE STIMULANT
Animal studies show that curcumin acts as a digestive stimulant and

encourages the release of digestive enzymes to start breaking down carbohydrate and fat.

● ANTI-INFLAMMATORY EFFECTS
Curcumin also has anti-inflammatory properties and inhibits platelet aggregation by influencing the formation of eicosanoids *(pp.22, 125)*.

TURMERIC: OTHER PHYTOCHEMICALS

FLAVONOIDS pp.34–35	
PHENOLIC ACIDS pp.56–57	

NUTRITIONAL VALUES
Quantities per 4oz.

CALORIES	354
FIBER	21g
POTASSIUM	2525mg
IRON	41mg

CRANBERRY

May reduce bladder infections ◆ Helps maintain a

healthy heart ◆ May have anti-inflammatory benefits

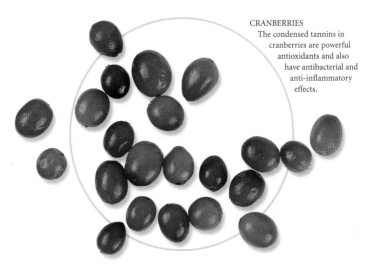

CRANBERRIES
The condensed tannins in
cranberries are powerful
antioxidants and also
have antibacterial and
anti-inflammatory
effects.

MAXIMIZING THE BENEFITS

An average portion of fresh cranberries weighs about 3oz. Frozen and dried cranberries and cranberry fruit juice are also available. Condensed tannins are not destroyed by cooking.

Note: most commercial cranberry products are also high in sugar.

HOW MUCH TO EAT

If prone to urinary tract infections, drinking 10oz. of cranberry juice daily may help or try eating a daily portion of cranberries.

KEY BENEFITS

Cranberries are a source of phytochemicals known as condensed tannins (or proanthocyanidins).

● URINARY TRACT INFECTIONS

Cranberry juice has long been recommended as a treatment for urinary tract infections. Recent scientific studies have identified condensed tannins as a key antibacterial factor. Cranberry juice may reduce the numbers of bacteria adhering to the urinary tract lining. A study of elderly women suggested a 50 percent reduction in infections in those who drank 10oz. cranberry juice daily over six months.

● HEART HEALTH

Condensed tannins are powerful antioxidants, and animal studies show they can inhibit the oxidation of "bad" LDL cholesterol and so protect against atherosclerosis. Condensed tannins are also found in red wine (and grape seeds), and are considered an important contributor to its heart-protective properties.

CRANBERRY: OTHER PHYTOCHEMICALS

FLAVONOIDS pp.34–35	
PHENOLIC ACIDS pp.56–57	

NUTRITIONAL VALUES
Quantities per 4oz.

CALORIES	15
FIBER	3g
VITAMIN C	13mg

RED WINE

Linked to a reduced risk of heart disease

Strong antioxidant effects

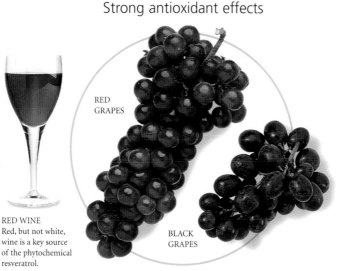

RED WINE
Red, but not white,
wine is a key source
of the phytochemical
resveratrol.

RED
GRAPES

BLACK
GRAPES

MAXIMIZING THE BENEFITS

The concentration of resveratrol in wine can vary according to the grapes used and where they are grown. Pinot noir grapes have especially high levels, and grapes grown in areas that provide warmth and some moisture, such as Burgundy, Bordeaux, and Chilean valleys, are optimal.

HOW MUCH TO DRINK

One 4 oz. glass per day may provide health benefits. Alcohol in wine promotes absorption of its unique phenolics.

KEY BENEFITS

Resveratrol is found in grape skins (where it acts as a natural fungicide for grapes), and hence red wine is a key source of this phytochemical. Red wine is famous for its heart health benefits, and its regular consumption may help explain the relatively low incidence of heart disease in France, despite high intakes of saturated fat. However, a moderate intake of any alcoholic drink has some heart-health benefits.

● **HEART DISEASE**
Studies reveal that resveratrol inhibits the oxidation of "bad" LDL cholesterol and platelet aggregation, so reducing the risk of atherosclerosis. Red wine contains other phenolics, too, and human studies show they are generally well-absorbed and increase antioxidant levels in the blood. Red wine has beneficial effects on "good" HDL cholesterol and helps to relax blood vessels (by increasing the release of nitric acid).

RED WINE: OTHER PHYTOCHEMICALS

CONDENSED TANNINS	p.67
FLAVONOIDS	pp.34–35
PHENOLIC ACIDS	pp.56–57

NUTRITIONAL VALUES
Quantities per 4oz.

CALORIES	70
POTASSIUM	110mg
IRON	0.9mg

PEANUT

Linked to a reduced risk of heart disease

Lowers cholesterol levels ◆ Has anticancer effects

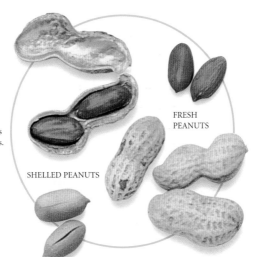

PEANUTS
Peanuts make a nutritious snack, or use in cooking. Peanut butter goes well in sandwiches.

FRESH PEANUTS

SHELLED PEANUTS

MAXIMIZING THE BENEFITS

Fresh peanuts in their shells are richest in resveratrol, vitamin E, and folate levels, and low in salt. Resveratrol levels are preserved in peanut butter. Nuts are high in calories, so in order to prevent weight gain, an increase in nut intake should be in place of other high-fat foods.

HOW MUCH TO EAT

Eating 1oz. of any type of nut (1tbsp. of peanut butter) at least five times a week has been linked to a 35% reduction in heart disease risk.

KEY BENEFITS

Peanuts are a key source of the phytochemical resveratrol, and regular nut consumption has been linked to a significant decrease in the risk of heart disease. Resveratrol also acts as a phyto-estrogen, which may help explain the health benefits of resveratrol-rich foods.

● HEART DISEASE
Resveratrol may protect against atherosclerosis. Peanuts also contain heart-healthy monounsaturated fat, vitamin E, folate, magnesium, potassium, selenium, saponins, and phytosterols. Moderate fat diets, with 50 percent of the fat content from

peanuts, can lower blood cholesterol levels as effectively as low-fat diets but without increasing levels of a type of fat – triglyceride – in the blood.

● CANCER
Animal studies indicate that resveratrol can inhibit the growth of damaged cells that lead to cancer.

PEANUT: OTHER PHYTOCHEMICALS

FLAVONOIDS	pp.34–35
PHYTOSTEROLS	p.97

NUTRITIONAL VALUES
Quantities per 4oz.

CALORIES	602
FIBER	6g
PROTEIN	25g
POTASSIUM	810mg
FOLATE	52mcg

CHILI PEPPERS

Eases nasal congestion ◆ Helps fight pain

Temporarily increases metabolic rate

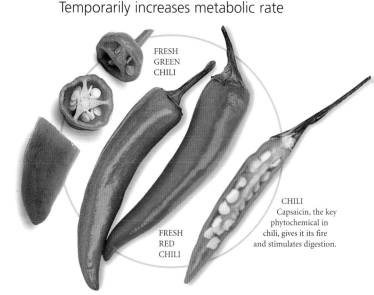

FRESH
GREEN
CHILI

CHILI
Capsaicin, the key
phytochemical in
chili, gives it its fire
and stimulates digestion.

FRESH
RED
CHILI

MAXIMIZING THE BENEFITS

The hotter the chili pepper, the higher the capsaicin content, which is concentrated mainly in the seeds and ribs, and the smaller the quantity needed. Personal preference will influence the choice of mild or hot chilies.

HOW MUCH TO EAT

A medium-sized chili weighs ¼oz. Chilies should not be consumed in large quantities; high consumers who repeatedly burn their mouth and stomach may increase their risk of developing cancer.

KEY BENEFITS

The key phytochemical in chili peppers is capsaicin, which helps to relieve nasal congestion. It also has antioxidant and anti-inflammatory effects.

● PAIN RELIEF

Skin creams containing capsaicin are clinically proven pain relievers. Psychologists suggest that the brain releases pain-killing and pleasure-giving endorphins in response to capsaicin's "heat," which may explain chili lovers' devotion to it.

● CANCER

Laboratory studies show capsaicin can inhibit cancer-causing agents and the growth of cancer cells, but also show it may promote cancer, although there is no solid evidence that moderate use promotes cancer.

● METABOLIC RATE

Eating chili may tempo-rarily raise the body's metabolic rate, but this should not be treated as a new slimming diet!

CHILI: OTHER PHYTOCHEMICALS

FLAVONOIDS	pp.34–35
CAROTENOIDS	pp.72–73

NUTRITIONAL VALUES
Quantities per 4oz

CALORIES	20
FIBER	1.6g
POTASSIUM	220mg
VITAMIN C	120mg

PARSLEY

Inhibits cancer-causing agents ◆ May have diuretic effects ◆ Good source of folate and vitamin C

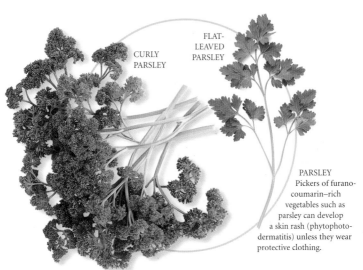

CURLY PARSLEY

FLAT-LEAVED PARSLEY

PARSLEY
Pickers of furano-coumarin–rich vegetables such as parsley can develop a skin rash (phytophoto-dermatitis) unless they wear protective clothing.

MAXIMIZING THE BENEFITS

Always use fresh parsley to maximize its folate and vitamin C benefits. Coumarins are not destroyed by cooking (they leach into cooking water) Tabbouleh is a classic parsley-rich dish, and its vitamin-C content boosts iron absorption from the parsley and cracked wheat.

HOW MUCH TO EAT

One tablespoon of parsley weighs ⅒oz. Herbalists recommend 1oz. a day for diuretic benefits but advise pregnant women to have ½oz. or less a day.

KEY BENEFITS

Parsley is a key source of coumarin phytochemicals. Coumarins affect blood-clotting mechanisms, and dicoumarin derivatives are used in anticoagulent drugs such as warfarin. Coumarins also have anti-oxidant activity. Enjoy parsley in salads, rice dishes, soups, sauces, and dressings. Fresh parsley also helps reduce breath odor from fresh garlic.

● DIURETIC

Parsley is reputed by herbalists to be a diuretic. It contains phthalides, a phytochemical also found in celery that has been reported to give celery a diuretic effect (p.124).

● CANCER

In laboratory studies coumarins inhibit the imitation of the development of cancer cells (p.19), and animal studies suggest this may be due their ability to stimulate enzymes that detoxify or block carcinogens.

PARSLEY: OTHER PHYTOCHEMICALS

| FLAVONOIDS pp.34–35 |
| PHENOLIC ACIDS pp.56–57 |
| CAROTENOIDS pp.72–73 |

NUTRITIONAL VALUES
Quantities per 4oz.

CALORIES	34
FIBER	5g
POTASSIUM	760mg
FOLATE	170mcg
VITAMIN C	190mg

GUIDE TO CAROTENOIDS

It is the phytochemicals known as carotenoids that make tomatoes red, corn yellow, and apricots orange. Like most other phytochemicals, carotenoids also appear to convey great health benefits.

Carotenoid phytochemicals help to keep plants healthy by working with the green pigment chlorophyll (p.106) to absorb sunlight for energy and growth. Conversely, if there is too much sunlight, carotenoids can switch roles and protect the plant by casting off this excess energy as heat. Carotenoids also work as antioxidants to mop up potentially damaging free radicals produced by exposure to ultraviolet light from sunlight. When we eat carotenoid-rich plants, we reap these anti-oxidant benefits, too.

THE BENEFITS OF CAROTENOIDS

In 1930 it was discovered that some colored plant extracts, later to be known as carotenoids, could be converted into vitamin A. Decades later, after diets rich in dark green, red, and yellow fruit and vegetables were consistently linked to a decreased risk in cancer, other potential benefits of carotenoids were recognized.

There are approximately 600 different carotenoids in plants, but only about 50 are found in the human diet, and only 20 or so have been identified in the body. Of these, six have so far been shown to play an important role in human health. These are alpha-carotene, beta-carotene, lycopene, lutein, cryptoxanthin, and zeaxanthin. It is also possible that unabsorbed carotenoids have "yet to be discovered" beneficial effects as they pass through the digestive tract.

All carotenoids are fat-soluble, meaning they need to be absorbed along with some fat in the diet. Once absorbed into the bloodstream, they are carried along in special proteins called lipoproteins (including low density lipoprotein, or LDL, that carries cholesterol around the blood). Like other phytochemicals, they don't appear to be essential to life, but high intakes are linked to a reduced risk of a variety of common disorders, for example, heart disease, cancers (particularly cancer of the lung, esophagus, stomach, colon, breast, and cervix), cataracts, Alzheimer's disease, dementia, and Type 2 diabetes. Research has also highlighted how carotenoids work as a team with each other and with antioxidant nutrients such as vitamin C. Single carotenoids, given as supplements, simply don't offer the same protection as combinations derived from food sources.

OTHER CHARACTERISTICS

In addition to preventing and controlling the generation of damaging free radicals, some carotenoids can be converted into vitamin A. They also play a role in maintaining the immune system, promoting healthy skin, preserving good vision, and inhibiting the development of cancer cells via cell-to-cell communication.

Excess vitamin A in the diet can be toxic, but eating carotenoid-rich fruit and vegetables regularly is safe for the body only converts as much vitamin A as it needs from carotenoids. However, very high intakes of carotenoids – from drinking a lot of carrot juice daily or taking more than 30mg supplements – may turn the skin an orange-yellow color, known as hypercarotenosis. This is a harmless condition, easily reversed by reducing the amount of carotenoid intake.

As with most phytochemicals, there are currently no recommended intakes for carotenoids. The general advice is to eat at least five portions of fruit and vegetables every day. Choosing deeply colored green and red-orange fruit and vegetables will enhance carotenoid intake. For example, broccoli, carrots, spinach, watermelon, tomatoes, and red peppers will provide optimal levels of carotenoids, whereas potatoes, apples, pears, onions, and eggplant provide few carotenoids. However, these foods are good sources of phenolics and a very important part of a health-promoting diet. Variety is the key to getting the phytochemical mix right.

GUIDE TO GOOD FOOD SOURCES OF CAROTENOIDS:

◆ **ALPHA-CAROTENE**
Carrots, pumpkins, avocados, tomatoes, corn, red peppers.

◆ **BETA-CAROTENE**
Carrots, red peppers, sweet potatoes, pumpkins, cantaloupes, apricots, cape gooseberries, endive, broccoli, mangos, kale, spinach, collard greens, parsley, rocket, watercress, basil, tamarillo, papayas.

◆ **LYCOPENE**
Tomatoes, pink grapefruit, watermelons, rosehips, guava, apricots.

◆ **LUTEIN**
Spinach, kale, spring/collard greens, broccoli, kiwifruit, Brussels sprouts, romaine lettuce, green peas, rhubarb, corn, yellow squash.

◆ **CRYPTOXANTHIN**
Papaya, persimmon, red peppers, tangerines, watermelon, mangos, tamarillo, guavas, nectarines, passion fruit, oranges.

◆ **ZEAXANTHIN**
Spinach, collard greens, corn, persimmons, romaine lettuce, tangerines.

BUTTERNUT SQUASH

Has anticancer effects ◆ May help preserve lung function

Useful source of vitamins A and C

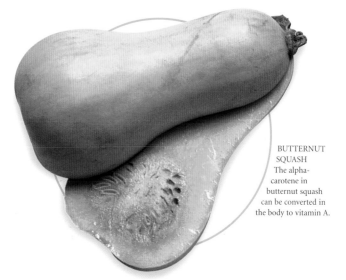

BUTTERNUT SQUASH
The alpha-carotene in butternut squash can be converted in the body to vitamin A.

MAXIMIZING THE BENEFITS

Alphacarotene is best absorbed when the pumpkin is cooked and eaten with fat, so make it part of a mixed meal or dish that contains a small amount of fat or oil.

HOW MUCH TO EAT

An average serving of baked butternut squash weighs 4oz. Bake or steam butternut squash as a vegetable, or cut in two, fill, and bake. It can also be puréed or used in soups or pumpkin pies, and to add moistness to fruit cakes and scones.

KEY BENEFITS

Butternut squash and pumpkin are rich sources of the phytochemical alphacarotene, which has antioxidant abilities and can inhibit cancer cell development.

● **CERVICAL CANCER**
Cervical dysplasia is the abnormal development of cells in the cervix and an early warning sign of cervical cancer. In a Japanese study of women with and without cervical dysplasia, those with higher blood levels of alphacarotene were significantly associated with a decreased risk of the disease after correcting for other risk factors.

● **LUNG FUNCTION**
A good antioxidant status may protect against the reduction in lung function over time. In a study of Dutch men aged 65 to 85 years, those with the highest blood levels of alphcarotene had significantly better lung function than those with the lowest levels.

SQUASH: OTHER PHYTOCHEMICALS

OTHER CAROTENOIDS pp.72–73	
FLAVONOIDS pp.34–35	

NUTRITIONAL VALUES
Quantities per 4oz., baked

CALORIES	32
FIBER	1.4g
POTASSIUM	280mg
VITAMIN C	15mg

AVOCADO

Good for heart health ◆ Has antioxidant ability

Source of vitamin E and potassium

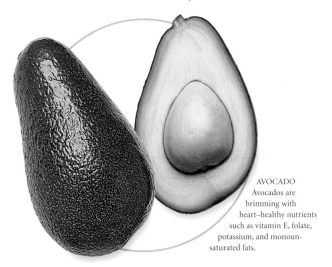

AVOCADO
Avocados are brimming with heart–healthy nutrients such as vitamin E, folate, potassium, and monoun-saturated fats.

MAXIMIZING THE BENEFITS

Alphacarotene is best absorbed with some fat, as is vitamin E. Avocado, a natural source of monoun-saturated fat, makes an ideal, self-contained heart-healthy food package. Avocados also provide vitamins B6 and C.

HOW MUCH TO EAT

Half a medium avocado (flesh only) weighs 2½oz. Serve with sliced fruit, tomato, or in salads, as guacomale, or puréed and baked in a pie. While nutritious, it is also high in calories, so moderate your intake.

KEY BENEFITS

Alpha-carotene is found in moderate amounts in avocados. Like other carotenoids, its anti-oxidant powers help it to protect against oxidation of "bad" LDL cholesterol in the body, so reducing the risk of atherosclerosis over time.

● ANGINA

Angina is the pain caused when blood flow to the heart is restricted by atherosclerosis. A study in the U.S. involving 11,300 people found that those with the highest blood levels of alphacarotene had a significantly lower risk compared to those with the lowest levels.

● ALZHEIMER'S DISEASE

Low antioxidant status may influence the develop-ment of Alzheimer's disease. A study found blood levels of alpha-carotene, but not vitamin E, to be significantly lower in people with the condition compared to people without it.

AVOCADO: OTHER PHYTOCHEMICALS

OTHER CAROTENOIDS	pp.72–73
PHENOLIC ACIDS	pp.56–57
BIOGENIC AMINES	p.104

NUTRITIONAL VALUES
Quantities per 4oz., flesh

CALORIES	190
FIBER	3.4g
POTASSIUM	450mg
VITAMIN E	3.2mg

CARROT

Linked to a reduced risk of lung cancer ◆ Stimulates

the immune system ◆ Useful for women on the pill

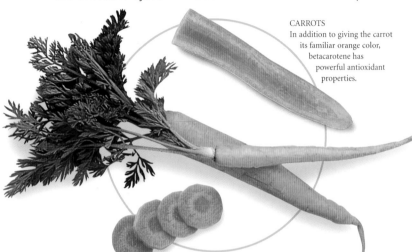

CARROTS
In addition to giving the carrot its familiar orange color, betacarotene has powerful antioxidant properties.

MAXIMIZING THE BENEFITS

Like all carotenoids, betacarotene is best absorbed by the body when eaten with a little oil or fat. Cooking carrots will also help in the absorption of some of its carotenoids.

HOW MUCH TO EAT

A medium carrot weighs 3oz. To increase blood-levels of beta-carotene and other carotenoids found in carrots, eat them as part of a dressed salad, in stir fries, casseroles, as a vegetable, or juiced and drunk with a meal.

KEY BENEFITS

Betacarotene is the principal phytochemical in carrots and can convert into vitamin A, which is important for healthy skin and eyes and for the immune system.

● LUNG CANCER

Eating carrots regularly may be linked to a reduced risk of lung cancer. A 16-year study of American female nurses found that women who ate five or more carrots a week had 60 percent lower risk of developing lung cancer than those who ate none.

● CONTRACEPTIVE PILL

Women taking the pill may benefit from a regular betacarotene intake, as a German study indicated that pill use may result in lower blood levels of betacarotene.

● NIGHT VISION

There is some truth in the saying that carrots help you see in the dark. Vitamin A helps protect against night blindness (poor vision in dim light).

CARROT: OTHER PHYTOCHEMICALS

| OTHER CAROTENOIDS pp.72–73 |
| FLAVONOIDS pp.34–35 |

NUTRITIONAL VALUES
Quantities per 4oz.

CALORIES	35
FIBER	2.4g
POTASSIUM	170mg
VITAMIN C	6mg

SWEET POTATO

Aids iron absorption from cereals ◆ Linked to
reduced risk of arthritis ◆ Source of vitamin E

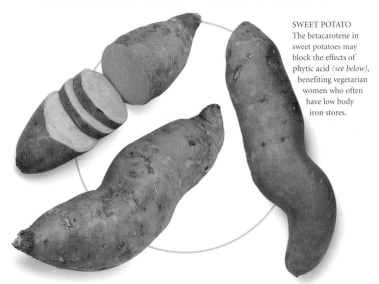

SWEET POTATO
The betacarotene in
sweet potatoes may
block the effects of
phytic acid *(see below)*,
benefiting vegetarian
women who often
have low body
iron stores.

MAXIMIZING THE BENEFITS

Sweet potatoes are a good source of alpha-carotene as well as betacarotene, which are best absorbed when eaten with fat (as is vitamin E), so eat as part of a meal. The deeper orange the sweet potato, the higher its beta-carotene content.

HOW MUCH TO EAT

An average portion of boiled sweet potatoes weighs 4–5oz. Sweet potatoes are also delicious baked, mashed, or as an ingredient in puréed vegetable soup.

KEY BENEFITS

Sweet potatoes are brimming with betacarotene. They also contain anti-oxidant vitamins C and E, which maximize the effectiveness of carotenoids as free radical fighters.

● **SKIN PROTECTION**
High blood levels of beta-carotene can reduce skin sensitivity to sunlight. This is not a substitute for sunscreen lotions and sun exposure precautions.

● **IRON ABSORPTION**
Betacarotene appears to double the rate of iron absorption from foods such as rice, corn, and wheat. It may do this by blocking the iron-binding effects of phytochemicals such as phytic acid *(p.111)* and phenolics, which reduce iron absorption.

● **ARTHRITIS**
Good levels of beta-carotene in the body have been linked to a reduced risk of developing rheumatoid arthritis. Low levels of antioxidants may be a risk factor.

SWEET POTATO: OTHER
PHYTOCHEMICALS

FLAVONOIDS	pp.34–35
PHENOLIC ACIDS	pp.56–57

NUTRITIONAL VALUES
Quantities per 4oz., boiled

CALORIES	84
FIBER	2.3g
POTASSIUM	300mg
VITAMIN E	4.4mg

TOMATO

Has anticancer effects ◆ Linked to a reduced risk of heart attack ◆ Useful source of vitamins C and E

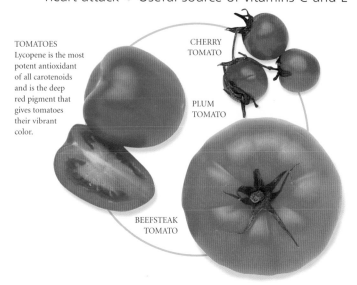

TOMATOES
Lycopene is the most potent antioxidant of all carotenoids and is the deep red pigment that gives tomatoes their vibrant color.

CHERRY TOMATO

PLUM TOMATO

BEEFSTEAK TOMATO

MAXIMIZING THE BENEFITS

For maximum absorption lycopene must be released from tomato cells; it is most easily absorbed from tomatoes that have been heat-processed in some way. A little oil or dressing also aids absorption. Cherry tomatoes are especially rich in flavonoids.

HOW MUCH TO EAT

A medium tomato weighs 3oz. Regularly eat tomatoes roasted, raw, or broiled, or use them as juice, purée, pulped (often sold as passata) – or even as tomato ketchup.

KEY BENEFITS

The main phytochemical present in tomatoes is lycopene. Up to 85 percent of lycopene in the diet comes from tomatoes and tomato products.

● **PROSTATE CANCER**
Lycopene is the main antioxidant in the prostate gland. A study of 47,000 American men showed that those who ate tomato products 10 or more times a week had 35 percent less risk of developing cancer. Risk reduction was also apparent with at least two tomato portions per week.

● **HEART DISEASE**
A study of European men showed that those with high levels of lycopene in their bodies had half the risk of heart attack as men with low levels.

● **CANCERS OF THE DIGESTIVE TRACT**
Trials suggest that a high intake of lycopene from tomatoes is linked to a reduced risk of cancers of the stomach, colon, and rectal cancers.

TOMATO: OTHER PHYTOCHEMICALS

FLAVONOIDS	pp.34–35
PHYTOSTEROLS	p.97

NUTRITIONAL VALUES
Quantities per 4oz.

CALORIES	17
FIBER	1g
VITAMIN C	17mg
VITAMIN E	1.2mg

PINK GRAPEFRUIT

Has anticancer effects ◆ May help people with diabetes
Good source of vitamin C

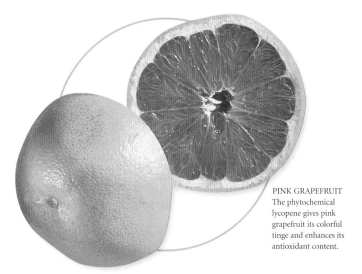

PINK GRAPEFRUIT
The phytochemical lycopene gives pink grapefruit its colorful tinge and enhances its antioxidant content.

MAXIMIZING THE BENEFITS

Make pink grapefruit part of a meal to help lycopene absorption into the body. As lycopene is optimally absorbed from heated foods, and grapefruit is usually eaten fresh, include other lycopene sources, too – for example, tomato sauce on pasta.

HOW MUCH TO EAT

Half a medium pink grapefruit weighs 6oz. Start the day with half a pink grapefruit or a glass of grapefruit juice with breakfast. Also add to green or rice salads, fruit salad, or fruit cocktails.

KEY BENEFITS

Once the lycopene in pink grapefruit has mopped up free radicals in the body, the vitamin C in the fruit can regenerate lycopene's antioxidant powers.

● **DIABETES**
People with diabetes generally produce large amounts of free radicals, which may increase their risk of heart disease, eye, and kidney problems; higher intakes of anti-oxidants may reduce the risk of these complications. An American study of 1,665 adults (aged 40 to 75) found that those with newly diagnosed diabetes or "impaired glucose tolerance" (which can lead to diabetes) had lower blood levels of lycopene and other carotenoids, compared to "healthy" people.

● **STROKE**
Eating citrus fruit as part of six or more portions of fruit and vegetables daily is linked to reduced risk of stroke.

GRAPEFRUIT: OTHER PHYTOCHEMICALS

OTHER CAROTENOIDS pp.72–73	
FLAVONOIDS pp.34–35	
PHENOLIC ACID pp.56–57	

NUTRITIONAL VALUES
Quantities per 4oz.

CALORIES	32
FIBER	1.1g
POTASSIUM	129mg
VITAMIN C	38mg

SPINACH

May protect against ARMD ◆ Linked a to reduced risk of colon cancer ◆ Good source of folate and vitamin E

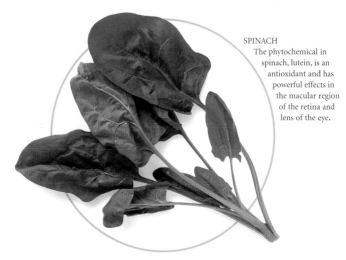

SPINACH
The phytochemical in spinach, lutein, is an antioxidant and has powerful effects in the macular region of the retina and lens of the eye.

MAXIMIZING THE BENEFITS

Eat spinach with a dressing or as part of a mixed meal, as lutein absorption is enhanced by fat. Cooking helps, too, but keep cooking times short to conserve the vitamin C and folate content.

HOW MUCH TO EAT

An average serving of cooked spinach weighs 3oz. Eat 5 servings of lutein-rich foods a week. Rinse and use spinach raw in salads, or sauté for 2-3 minutes. Spinach goes well with yogurt or feta cheese. It can also accumulate nitrates from the soil (see p.109).

KEY BENEFITS

Spinach is an important source of the phyto-chemical lutein, which works with its partner carotenoid zeaxanthin to protect against age-related deterioration of vision.

● ARMD

Age-related macular degeneration (ARMD) is the most common cause of blindness in the West. A study in the U.S. found people who ate spinach or leafy greens (5 servings or more a week), had a 43 percent lower risk of developing ARMD com-pared to those who ate the least. Eating spinach regularly may improve vision for some sufferers.

● COLON CANCER

An American study examining the link between carotenoid intake and colon cancer concluded that regularly eating lutein-rich foods, especially spinach, may help reduce the risk of developing this cancer.

SPINACH: OTHER PHYTOCHEMICALS

OTHER CAROTENOIDS	pp.72–73
CHLOROPHYLL	p.106
PHENOLIC ACIDS	pp.56–57
PHYTOSTEROLS	p.97

NUTRITIONAL VALUES
Quantities per 4oz., boiled

CALORIES	21
FIBER	2.1g
FOLATE	90mcg
VITAMIN E	1.7mg
POTASSIUM	340mg

KALE

Helps reduce risk of cataracts ◆ Linked to a reduced risk of cancers ◆ Good source calcium and folate

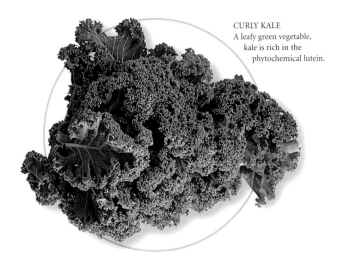

CURLY KALE
A leafy green vegetable, kale is rich in the phytochemical lutein.

MAXIMIZING THE BENEFITS

Fat promotes the absorption of lutein and other carotenoids in kale, so serve cooked as part of a meal. Kale is also an excellent source of calcium that is well absorbed by the body (unlike the calcium in spinach due to its oxalate content, p.111).

HOW MUCH TO EAT

An average portion of kale weighs 3oz. Enjoy kale in gratin dishes or stir fries, or simply steamed. A little vegetable broth and butter or margarine adds extra flavor.

KEY BENEFITS

Kale ranks as having the highest overall antioxidant ability (p.25) of leafy green vegetables, and is a good source of protective lutein, other carotenoids, folate, vitamins C and E, and glucosinolates (p.90).

● CATARACTS
Lutein is present in the lens of the eye. Excess free radical damage in the lens can result in cataracts. Two American studies of the diet and health of 100,000 men and women revealed that those with the highest intakes of lutein-rich foods had a 20 percent reduced risk of cataract extraction, compared to those with the lowest intakes.

● CANCER
Numerous population studies have linked regular intakes of leafy green vegetables such as kale to a reduced risk of cancers at different sites in the body, in particular cancers of the colon, mouth, stomach, lung, and breast.

KALE: OTHER PHYTOCHEMICALS

| OTHER CAROTENOIDS pp.72–73 |
| FLAVONOIDS pp.34–35 |
| GLUCOSINOLATES pp.90–91 |

NUTRITIONAL VALUES
Quantities per 4oz., boiled

CALORIES	24
FIBER	2.8g
CALCIUM	150mg
FOLATE	86mcg
VITAMIN C	71mg

MANGO & PAPAYA

Linked to a reduced risk of cervical cancer
and colon cancer ◆ Good source of vitamins C and E

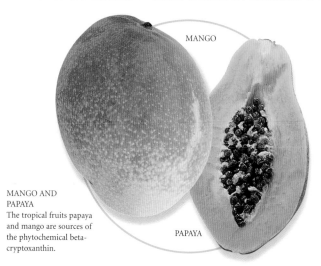

MANGO

PAPAYA

MANGO AND PAPAYA
The tropical fruits papaya and mango are sources of the phytochemical beta-cryptoxanthin.

MAXIMIZING THE BENEFITS

Beta-cryptoxanthin is best absorbed when eaten with fat, so to maximize benefit try to eat mangos or papaya as part of a mixed meal rather than on their own.

HOW MUCH TO EAT

An average mango (flesh only) or slice of papaya weighs around 6oz. To increase levels of beta-cryptoxanthin (and the betacarotene they contain) in the body, add to mixed or fruit salads, or on cereals. They also taste delicious in smoothies and juices, or as salsa.

KEY BENEFITS

The phytochemical beta-cryptoxanthin in papaya and mango has protective antioxidant properties and can be converted by the body into vitamin A.

● CANCER

A study by New Zealand researchers was conducted to help them understand differences in the rates of colon cancer between Poly-nesians and Europeans living in New Zealand. Mango and papaya were identified as foods with cancer-fighting properties often eaten by Polynesians.

● CERVICAL CANCER

A carotenoid-rich diet may reduce the risk of cervical cancer. A 15-year study of 15,000 women established a link between high intakes of cryptoxanthin-rich food and a significantly reduced risk of cervical cancer. Similar associations were found for the other carotenoids that can be converted to vitamin A – alphacarotene and betacarotene.

MANGO: OTHER PHYTOCHEMICALS

OTHER CAROTENOIDS	pp.72–73
PHENOLIC ACIDS	pp.56–57

NUTRITIONAL VALUES
Quantities per 4oz., mango

CALORIES	57
FIBER	2.6g
VITAMIN C	37mg
VITAMIN E	1mg

RED PEPPER

Linked to reduced risk of heart disease

High antioxidant content ◆ Excellent source of vitamin C

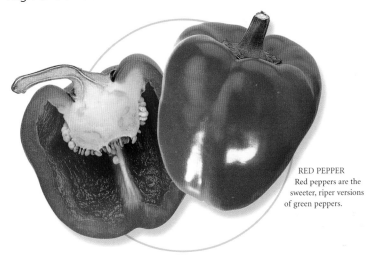

RED PEPPER
Red peppers are the
sweeter, riper versions
of green peppers.

MAXIMIZING THE BENEFITS

Beta-cryptoxanthin, vitamin E, and other carotenoids in peppers are best absorbed when eaten with some oil, so eat as part of a mixed meal.

HOW MUCH TO EAT

Half a red pepper weighs 3oz. Use sliced in salads, stir fries, pasta sauces, and Mexican dishes, or stuff a whole, deribbed pepper and bake. Red peppers contain the most beta-cryptoxanthin, but yellow and green varieties contain other carotenoids, especially betacarotene.

KEY BENEFITS

Red peppers are an excellent source of the phytochemical beta-cryptoxanthin, and also betacarotene. The exceptional vitamin C content of a red pepper helps to regenerate and enhance the protective effects of its carotenoids, which act as antioxidants in the body.

● **HEART DISEASE**
High blood levels of beta-cryptoxanthin have been associated with a reduced risk of angina. Further heart health links were highlighted by a study that compared the blood levels of nutrients and phytochemicals of people in Toulouse, France (where heart disease rates are low), and Belfast, Northern Ireland (where rates are high). The major differences were carotenoid levels: blood levels of beta-cryptoxanthin were twice as high in the Toulouse population (as were lutein levels).

RED PEPPER: OTHER
PHYTOCHEMICALS

OTHER CAROTENOIDS	pp.72–73
FLAVONOIDS	pp.34–35
CAPSAICIN	p.70

NUTRITIONAL VALUES
Quantities per 4oz.

CALORIES	32
FIBER	1.6g
FOLATE	21mcg
VITAMIN C	140mg
VITAMIN E	0.8mg

ROMAINE LETTUCE

Helps protect against ARMD ◆ Linked to a reduced

risk of cancers ◆ Good source of folate

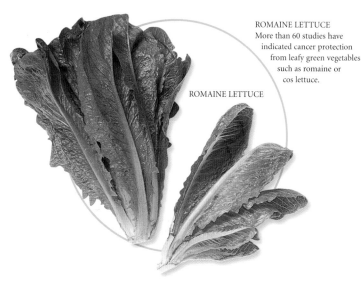

ROMAINE LETTUCE
More than 60 studies have
indicated cancer protection
from leafy green vegetables
such as romaine or
cos lettuce.

ROMAINE LETTUCE

MAXIMIZING THE BENEFITS

The dark, outer leaves of romaine lettuce are richest in carotenoids. Zeaxanthin is best absorbed when eaten with a little oil, so eat with a dressing or as part of a meal. Store in the fridge and use fresh to make the most of its folate and vitamin C content.

HOW MUCH TO EAT

Four large leaves weigh about 3oz. Rinse well and use as a garnish and in salads; it is most famous as an ingredient for Caesar salad. It also accumulates nitrates from the soil (p.109).

KEY BENEFITS

Romaine lettuce is an important source of the antioxidant phyto-chemical zeaxanthin. It also contains lutein, a carotenoid that works closely with zeaxanthin to help protect against age-related visual problems.

● ARMD

Zeaxanthin and lutein are the only carotenoids found in the macular pigment, which helps form the macular (responsible for detailed vision) found in the center of the retina. This pigment helps filter free radical-generating wavelengths of light. Working as antioxidants, zeaxanthin and lutein

may help protect the macular from free radical damage, so reducing the risk of ARMD.

● CANCER

Zeaxanthin, alongside vitamin C, lutein, beta-carotene, folate, and flavonols in green vegetables such as lettuce all contribute to their cancer-protective effects.

LETTUCE: OTHER PHYTOCHEMICALS

| OTHER CAROTENOIDS | pp.72–73 |
| FLAVONOIDS | pp.34–35 |

NUTRITIONAL VALUES
Quantities per 4oz.

CALORIES	16
FIBER	1.2g
POTASSIUM	220mg
FOLATE	55mcg

CORN

Fights free radicals in the retina

Helps protect against ARMD ◆ Good source of folate

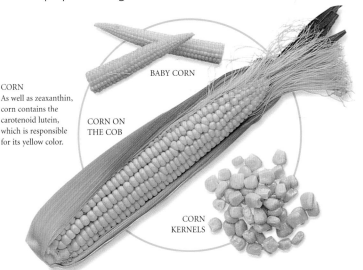

BABY CORN

CORN
As well as zeaxanthin, corn contains the carotenoid lutein, which is responsible for its yellow color.

CORN ON THE COB

CORN KERNELS

MAXIMIZING THE BENEFITS

Zeaxanthin is best absorbed along with some fat; cooking corn will also boost absorption. Delicate baby corn is notably high in folate, so keep cooking times short to conserve folate levels.

HOW MUCH TO EAT

A portion of corn kernels weighs 3oz. Also enjoy corn straight from the cob. Baby corn is best in stir fries. Make popcorn by cooking dried kernels in a frying pan with a lid securely on and shaking regularly.

KEY BENEFITS

Corn is a prime source of the antioxidant phytochemical zeaxanthin. Together with another antioxidant carotenoid, lutein, zeaxanthin may help to reduce ARMD.

● ANTIOXIDANT EFFECTS IN THE EYE
Research shows that lutein and zeaxanthin are found in highest concentrations in the part of the retina that contains most of the lipids susceptible to free radical attack and damage.

● ARMD
When 6oz. corn with and without 2oz. of spinach was eaten daily for four weeks by people with ARMD, blood levels of carotenoids increased for most. In addition, the density of their macular pigment increased and remained this way for several months. Increased macular pigment density helps filter and protect the eye from damaging wavelengths of light.

CORN: OTHER PHYTOCHEMICALS

PHENOLIC ACIDS	pp.56–57
PHYTOSTEROLS	p.97
FRUCTO-OLIGOSACCHARIDES	pp.98–99

NUTRITIONAL VALUES
Quantities per 4oz., boiled

CALORIES	111
FIBER	2.2g
FOLATE	34mcg
POTASSIUM	240mg

GUIDE TO OTHER KEY PHYTOCHEMICALS

There are of thousands of "other" phytochemicals, but only a relatively small number have been isolated and investigated for their potential effects on health. This section highlights the best studied phytochemicals and their food sources.

Garlic, that famous "healing food," kicks off this final phytochemical collection. Its health benefits have been recognized for thousands of years, not to mention its vampire-scaring abilities. Despite this, there are still many unanswered questions about how garlic's sulfur-based phytochemicals work in the body, what happens when we cook garlic, and how much we need to eat.

Garlic supplements abound, and it may be that they have useful therapeutic effects – lowering blood pressure or cholesterol, for example. However, they currently vary so much in form, dosage, and quality of research that it still makes sense to look to your overall diet first. Eating a diet rich in a variety of plant foods and enjoying garlic's unique pungency in your cooking is the best way to reap benefits.

OTHER PLANT FOODS

Cruciferous vegetables, commonly known as the cabbage family, are also part of this category. These mostly green leafy vegetables are oozing with goodness and health-promoting phytochemicals.

Unfortunately, the very phyto-chemicals that seem so good for us can also taste bitter to some people (they were no doubt much more bitter growing in the wild, to deter any predators).

Special forms of dietary fiber, fructo-oligosaccharides, are also discussed in this section. While not strictly phytochemicals, they do appear to have uniquely beneficial effects on health over and above helping to keep us regular.

Some of the reported health effects of a number of phytochemicals highlighted in *Super Nutrients* have been achieved with greater amounts of phytochemicals than we can get simply by eating plant foods. This research helps to build our under-standing of how phytochemicals function and direct scientists toward the next stage of research. This will increasingly involve trials of people eating reasonable amounts of a variety of plant foods. It is encouraging to remember that population studies show that standard fruit and vegetable-rich diets do help protect people's health, and that they don't need artificially high intakes of phytochemicals or nutrients to achieve these benefits. The Mediterranean diet *(p.14)* is a great example of this and shows just how the overall package of a healthy diet can nourish body, mind, and soul.

OTHER KEY PHYTO-CHEMICALS AND THEIR FOOD SOURCES:

◆ **ALLIUM COMPOUNDS, E.G., ALLYLIC SULFIDES**
Garlic, onions, leeks, scallions, chives.

◆ **DITHIOLTHIONES & GLUCOSINOLATES, E.G., ISOTHIOCYANATES, INDOLES**
Cruciferous vegetables – broccoli, cabbage, Brussels sprouts, kale, kohlrabi – mustard greens, horseradish, watercress, turnip greens.

◆ **PROTEASE INHIBITORS**
Barley, wholewheat foods, oats, rye, soy beans, kidney beans, garbanzo beans, lentils.

◆ **PHYTIC ACID**
Bran, wholewheat foods, sesame seeds, lima beans, peanuts, soy beans, almonds, black beans, haricot beans, string beans, lentils.

◆ **PHYTOSTEROLS, E.G., BETA SITOSTEROL, CAMPOSTEROL, STIGMASTEROL**
Soy beans, wheatgerm, buckwheat, sesame seeds, rye, corn, sunflower seeds, pumpkin seeds, peanuts, oats, basil, eggplant.

◆ **FRUCTO-OLIGOSACCHARIDES**
Jerusalem artichokes, bananas, endive, leeks, onions, wholewheat foods, asparagus, sunflower seeds, corn, cucumbers, peas, garbanzo beans, alfalfa sprouts.

◆ **FUCOXANTHINS & AGAR AGAR**
Seaweed.

◆ **LENTINAN**
Shiitake mushrooms.

◆ **MONOTERPENES, E.G., LIMONENE**
Citrus fruit (pith, peel, and juice), celery, caraway seeds, cherries, herbs.

◆ **LIMONOIDS**
Citrus fruit (pith, peel, and juice).

◆ **SAPONINS**
Alfalfa sprouts, garbanzo beans, soy beans, mung bean sprouts, quinoa, kidney beans, peanuts, climbing beans, oats, tomatoes, asparagus.

◆ **BIOGENIC AMINES, E.G., SEROTONIN, DOPAMINE, PHENYLETHYLAMINE**
Plantains, bananas, kiwifruit, pineapples, walnuts, grapes, pecans, apples, avocados, broccoli, Brussels sprouts, cocoa beans, Chinese mushrooms, wine.

◆ **XANTHINE ALKALOIDS**
Caffeine (coffee, tea, cocoa, cola drinks), theobromine (cocoa, coffee), theophylline (tea).

◆ **PLANT ENZYMES, E.G., BROMELAIN, PAPAIN, ACTINIDIN**
Pineapples, papaya, kiwifruit.

GARLIC

Promotes heart health ◆ Has anticancer effects

Has antibacterial effects

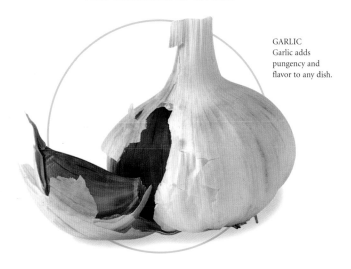

GARLIC
Garlic adds
pungency and
flavor to any dish.

MAXIMIZING THE BENEFITS

When garlic is crushed or chewed, the enzyme allinase is released and converts the allylic sulfide (alliin) to the pungent allicin. Allicin then breaks down into more sulfur compounds. Let crushed garlic stand for 10 minutes before cooking to preserve its beneficial compounds.

HOW MUCH TO EAT

One clove of garlic weighs ⅙oz. Beneficial health effects have been reported from eating between half to three or more cloves a day.

KEY BENEFITS

Garlic is a key source of phytochemicals known as allylic sulfides. Garlic has long had a strong reputation as a food that can help improve many common ailments.

● **ANTIBACTERIAL EFFECT**
Garlic is used as an antibacterial, antiviral, and antifungal agent in countries where modern medicines are scarce.

● **COLON CANCER**
Animal studies indicate that the allylic sulfides in garlic may help fight cancer by stimulating enzymes that detoxify cancer-causing agents in the gut.

● **HEART HEALTH**
There is conflicting evidence as to whether fresh garlic or supplements can lower cholesterol levels. Studies indicate a beneficial effect of garlic and garlic extracts on blood pressure and blood clotting. Garlic's phytochemicals also inhibit the oxidation of "bad" LDL cholesterol and so may reduce the risk of atherosclerosis.

GARLIC: OTHER PHYTOCHEMICALS

FLAVONOIDS pp.34–35

NUTRITIONAL VALUES
Quantities per 4oz.

CALORIES	98
FIBER	4.1g

LEEK

Linked to a reduced risk of heart disease

Has anticancer effects ◆ Useful source of folate and fiber

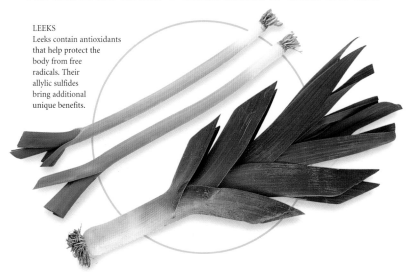

LEEKS
Leeks contain antioxidants that help protect the body from free radicals. Their allylic sulfides bring additional unique benefits.

MAXIMIZING THE BENEFITS

Leeks are not as rich in allylic sulfides as garlic or onions – but all contribute to the benefits of these sulfur compounds. Cooking appears to increase the level of some and reduce others. Leeks and onions also contain beneficial fructo-oligosaccharides *(p.98)*, which may also cause flatulence.

HOW MUCH TO EAT

An average serving of cooked leeks weighs 3oz. Enjoy in casseroles, soups, steamed, or in stir fries. Or serve with pasta and cheese sauce.

KEY BENEFITS

Leeks and other onions are a source of sulfur-containing phyto-chemicals called allylic sulfides.

● **HEART HEALTH**
A regular intake of onions and leeks has been linked to a reduced risk of heart disease and stroke in population studies. Phyto-chemicals such as allylic sulfides and flavonols *(p.42)* may contribute to this effect as both display antioxidant activity and beneficial effects on the circulation.

● **STOMACH CANCER**
Eleven studies linked a regular intake of foods rich in allylic sulfides with a reduced risk of the cancer. Allylic sulfides have been shown to induce enzymes that detoxify cancer-causing agents, and may also reduce the risk of this cancer by blocking the conversion of nitrate (found in foods) to nitrosamines *(p.109)*.

LEEK: OTHER PHYTOCHEMICALS

FLAVONOIDS pp.34–35
FRUCTO-OLIGOSACCHARIDES pp.98–99

NUTRITIONAL VALUES
Quantities per 4oz., boiled

CALORIES	21
FIBER	1.7g
FOLATE	40mcg
VITAMIN E	0.8mg

BROCCOLI

Has anticancer effects ◆ Packed with beneficial

phytochemicals ◆ Source of folate and vitamin C

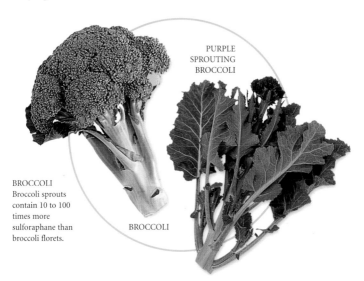

PURPLE
SPROUTING
BROCCOLI

BROCCOLI
Broccoli sprouts
contain 10 to 100
times more
sulforaphane than
broccoli florets.

BROCCOLI

MAXIMIZING THE BENEFITS

Cutting or chewing broccoli disrupts its cell walls and releases the enzyme myrosinase, which converts glucosinolates into the active sulforaphane. Steam or boil briefly to help conserve sulforaphane and vitamin levels.

HOW MUCH TO EAT

An average serving of two spears weighs 3–4oz. Enjoy fresh raw broccoli (or sprouts) in salads or as crudite for dips; or use in stir fries, in soups, pasta sauces, or as a vegetable.

KEY BENEFITS

Broccoli is an excellent source of the phytochemical sulforaphane; a type of isothiocyanate (derived from glucosinolates). It can inhibit the action of cancercausing agents by stimulating "phase two enzymes," one of the body's detoxification systems.

● CANCER

The cancer-fighting abilities of sulforaphane may help to explain studies that link regular intakes of cruciferous vegetables such as broccoli to a reduced risk of cancer, in particular of the bowel, stomach, breast, lungs, and kidneys.

● SUPER BROCCOLI

Researchers from the Institute of Food Research in Britain have recently bred a "super broccoli" – cultivated broccoli crossed with a wild relative – that has much higher levels of sulforaphane. It is not yet approved for sale.

BROCCOLI: OTHER PHYTOCHEMICALS

INDOLES AND DITHIOLTHIONES pp.92–93
CAROTENOIDS pp.72–73
FLAVONOIDS pp.34–35
LIGNANS pp.54–55

NUTRITIONAL VALUES

Quantities per 4oz., boiled

CALORIES	24
FIBER	2.4g
FOLATE	65mcg
VITAMIN C	44mg

BRUSSELS SPROUTS

Have anticancer effects ◆ Have many beneficial

phytochemicals ◆ Source of folate, vitamin C, and iron

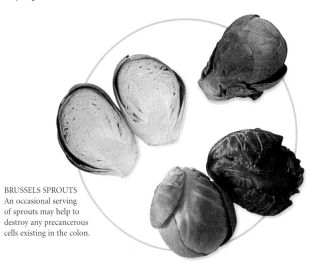

BRUSSELS SPROUTS
An occasional serving
of sprouts may help to
destroy any precancerous
cells existing in the colon.

MAXIMIZING THE BENEFITS

Cutting or chewing sprouts releases the enzyme myrosinase, which converts gluco- sinolates into sinigrin. After cooking (which destroys myrosinase), bacteria in the gut help take over this role. Steam or boil lightly to preserve the folate and vitamin C.

HOW MUCH TO EAT

Nine sprouts – an aver- age serving – weighs 3–4oz.; ¼lb. daily has been shown to reduce free radical damage in the body. Use as a side vegetable, in stir fries, or with chestnuts.

KEY BENEFITS

Brussels sprouts contain the phytochemical sinigrin, which is a type of isothiocyanate (derived from glucosinolates). This gives sprouts their distinc- tive smell and taste. People who inherit a tendency that makes certain chemicals taste bitter tend to also dislike sprouts! The challenge for food scientists is to breed a sprout that will maximize health bene- fits and please taste buds.

● **COLON CANCER**
Studies show that sinigrin exerts its cancer-fighting effects by triggering pre- cancerous cells to die (a naturally occurring process known as apoptosis). This

effect is so powerful that the occasional meal of sprouts could destroy pre- cancerous cells in the colon. Like other cruciferous vegetables, regular intakes are linked to reduced risk of a range of cancers.

BRUSSELS SPROUTS: OTHER PHYTOCHEMICALS

INDOLES AND DITHIOLTHIONES	pp.92–93
CAROTENOIDS	pp.72–73
FLAVONOIDS	pp.34–35
BIOGENIC AMINES	p.104

NUTRITIONAL VALUES
Quantities per 4oz., boiled

CALORIES	35
FIBER	3.1g
FOLATE	100mcg
VITAMIN C	60mg

GREEN CABBAGE

Has anticancer effects ◆ Traditional relief

for stomach ulcers ◆ Source of vitamin C and folate

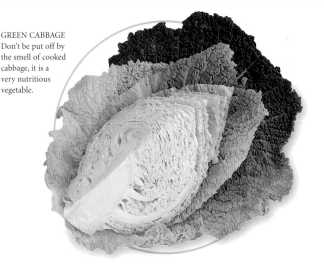

GREEN CABBAGE
Don't be put off by
the smell of cooked
cabbage, it is a
very nutritious
vegetable.

MAXIMIZING THE BENEFITS

Cutting or chewing cabbage releases the enzyme myrosinase, allowing the conversion of the glucosinolate "glucobrassin" into active indoles. Vitamin C helps form another type of indole, and cooking cabbage briefly helps conserve the required vitamin C.

HOW MUCH TO EAT

An average serving of cabbage weighs 4oz. Cabbage is versatile: use shredded in salads, soups, casseroles, or stir fries; whole leaves make baked cabbage parcels or a steamed vegetable.

KEY BENEFITS

Cabbage, a close relative of broccoli, is a key source of the glucosinolate-derived phytochemicals indoles. Indoles have anti-cancer activities, and 38 studies have linked diets rich in cabbage and other cruciferous vegetables with a reduced risk of a range of cancers.

● **CANCER**
Laboratory and animal studies suggest indoles may help fight cancer and block cancer-causing agents by stimulating "phase one" and "phase two" enzymes, both part of the body's detox-ification systems. They may also help reduce the exposure of breast cells to natural estrogen (high estrogen exposure can stimulate growth of breast cancer cells).

● **STOMACH ULCERS**
Drinking one quart of cabbage juice daily for eight days is a traditional remedy for pain relief and healing of stomach ulcers.

CABBAGE: OTHER PHYTOCHEMICALS

DITHIOLTHIONES	p.93
CAROTENOIDS	pp.72–73
FLAVONOIDS	pp.34–35

NUTRITIONAL VALUES
Quantities per 4oz., boiled

CALORIES	17
FIBER	2g
FOLATE	39mcg
VITAMIN C	19mg

BOK CHOI

Has anticancer effects ◆ Provides calcium

for bone health ◆ Source of folate and potassium

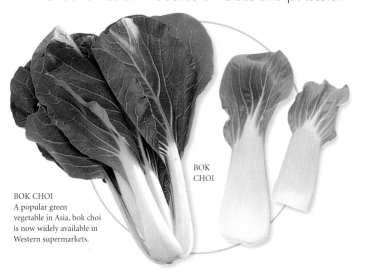

BOK
CHOI

BOK CHOI
A popular green
vegetable in Asia, bok choi
is now widely available in
Western supermarkets.

MAXIMIZING THE BENEFITS

Stir frying is an ideal cooking method to help conserve vitamin C and folate levels. If boiled, some calcium (and other minerals) can leach into cooking water. Whenever possible, use vegetable cooking water for soups and gravy – it contains lost minerals and phytochemicals.

HOW MUCH TO EAT

An average serving of bok choi weighs 4oz. It is a key ingredient for Asian dishes and adds a deliciously light, crunchy texture to soups, stir fries, and noodle dishes.

KEY BENEFITS

Bok choi is a source of sulfur-containing dithiolthione phyto-chemicals. Like other cruciferous vegetables, it also contains indoles and isothiocyanates.

● CALCIUM
Bok choi, along with kale, is a good source of calcium. Its flavonoid, vitamin, and mineral content makes it helpful overall for bone health.

● CANCER
Studies link regular intakes of cruciferous vegetables such as bok choi with a reduced risk of a number of cancers. Dithiolthiones may help

reduce the risk of cancer by stimulating "phase two" enzymes, which are part of the body's detoxi-fication system and can block the action of cancer-causing agents. Carotenoids in bok choi act as antioxidants so may reduce free radical damage in the body.

BOK CHOI: OTHER PHYTOCHEMICALS

| ISOTHIOCYANATES, INDOLES pp.90–92 |
| CAROTENOIDS pp.72–73 |
| FLAVONOIDS pp.34–35 |

NUTRITIONAL VALUES
Quantities per 4oz., cooked

CALORIES	12
FIBER	1.6g
CALCIUM	80mg
FOLATE	40mg

BARLEY AND RYE

Have anticancer effects ◆ May help reduce the risk

of heart disease ◆ Good source of soluble fiber

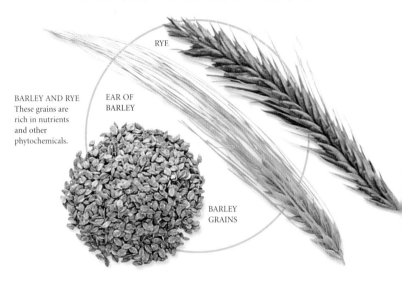

RYE

BARLEY AND RYE
These grains are
rich in nutrients
and other
phytochemicals.

EAR OF
BARLEY

BARLEY
GRAINS

MAXIMIZING THE BENEFITS

Pot barley or flakes are more nutritious than refined pearl barley. Barley and rye's soluble fiber content also helps regulate appetite and blood glucose levels.

HOW MUCH TO EAT

An average portion is 2 tbs. of barley (or flakes), 1 slice of heavy rye bread or 3 crispbread, of which three or more helpings daily could help reduce the risk of heart disease and cancer by 30%. Use barley as an alternative to rice. Sprinkle barley flakes on cereal and yogurt.

KEY BENEFITS

Barley and rye contain phytochemicals known as protease inhibitors, which have anticancer effects.

● **CANCER**
Proteases (enzymes) in cancer cells may enhance the cell's ability to invade surrounding healthy cells and spread cancer. Studies show that protease inhibitors can block the action of proteases and inhibit cancers. It is still uncertain as to how well plant protease inhibitors are absorbed and affect human proteases.

● **HEART DISEASE**
A six-year study of 22,000 Finnish men found that those who ate 1oz. fiber a day had 31 percent less chance of heart disease than those who ate 1oz. fiber. Much of this fiber came from wholegrain breads rich in rye, barley and oats. These grains are good sources of soluble fiber, other phyto-chemicals, and nutrients (vitamin E, magnesium, selenium, folate).

BARLEY: OTHER PHYTOCHEMICALS

PHENOLIC ACIDS	pp.56–57
PHYTOESTROGENS	pp.48–49
LIGNANS	pp.54–55

NUTRITIONAL VALUES
Quantities per 4oz., barley

CALORIES	301
FIBER	14.8g
POTASSIUM	560mg

OATS

Have anticancer effects ◆ Helps lower blood cholesterol

Useful source of magnesium and zinc

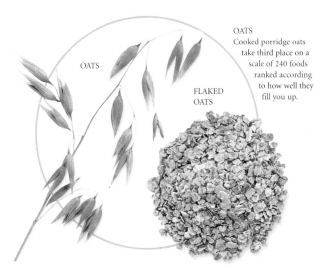

OATS

OATS
Cooked porridge oats take third place on a scale of 240 foods ranked according to how well they fill you up.

FLAKED OATS

MAXIMIZING THE BENEFITS

Oats can be eaten raw in granola or cooked as oatmeal, flapjacks, cobbler toppings; or use to bind foods like fishcakes or meatballs, or to thicken casseroles and soups.

HOW MUCH TO EAT

For an optimal cholesterol-lowering effect. 5 tbs. oats daily is recommended. But a more practical medium-large bowl of oatmeal daily brings health benefits, too. Two tablespoons of oats makes a medium bowl of oatmeal.

KEY BENEFITS

Like other wholegrains, oats are a source of the phytochemical phytic acid.

● CANCER
Laboratory and animal studies show that phytic acid has a range of anti-cancer effects *(see p.96)*.

● CHOLESTEROL LEVELS
Eating oats daily can result in modest cholesterol-lowering effects, and regulated health claims to this effect are permitted on oat products in the U.S. Beta-glucan, a type of spongelike soluble fiber, attracts cholesterol-based bile acids in the intestine and carries them out of the body. Cholesterol is

then pulled from the blood to make more bile acids, and so cholesterol levels are lowered.

● APPETITE
Foods rich in soluble fiber help regulate blood glucose levels and appetite, which can benefit weight control, heart disease, and diabetes.

OATS: OTHER PHYTOCHEMICALS

| PHENOLIC ACIDS pp.56–57 |
| PHYTOSTEROLS p.97 |
| PROTEASE INHIBITORS p.94 |

NUTRITIONAL VALUES
Quantities per 4oz.

CALORIES	401
FIBER	6.8g
MAGNESIUM	110mg
ZINC	3.3mg
VITAMIN E	1.5mg

SESAME SEEDS

Have anticancer effects ◆ Helps protect the body from

free radicals ◆ Source of magnesium and calcium

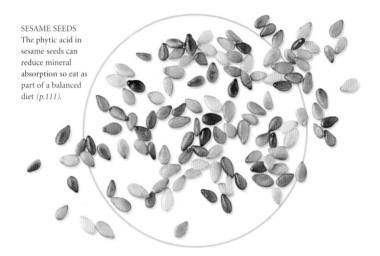

SESAME SEEDS
The phytic acid in sesame seeds can reduce mineral absorption so eat as part of a balanced diet *(p.111)*.

MAXIMIZING THE BENEFITS

Phytic acid is found in the outer layers of seeds, grains, and legumes, so eating whole seeds or grains maximizes the intake. Roasting sesame seeds gives the best flavor; cooking destroys unwanted phytochemicals.

HOW MUCH TO EAT

One tablespoon weighs ⅜oz. Use roasted seeds in baking, breakfast cereals, salads, and rice dishes, and as an ingredient in tahini, hummus, and falafel. Roasted sesame oil is widely used in Japanese and Chinese cooking.

KEY BENEFITS

Sesame seeds are a key source of phytic acid, which is found in the fibrous part of seeds, wholegrains, and legumes.

● BOWEL CANCER

Laboratory and animal studies suggest that phytic acid can inhibit cancer of the colon by acting as an antioxidant, decreasing the rate at which cancer cells spread and enhancing the immune system. Wholegrains are also rich in phytic acid, which may help explain their protective effects on colon cancer.

● MINERAL ABSORPTION

Phytic acid can bind and reduce the availability of minerals such as iron. This may be of benefit since excess iron in the intestine can increase free radicals.

● ANTIOXIDANTS

Sesame oil has strong antioxidant activity due to sesaminol, a lignan phytochemical *(pp.54–55)*, which is heat-stable.

SESAME SEEDS: OTHER PHYTOCHEMICALS

PHENOLIC ACIDS	pp.56–57
PHYTOSTEROLS	p.97
LIGNANS	pp.54–55

NUTRITIONAL VALUES
Quantities per 4oz

CALORIES	598
FIBER	7.9g
MAGNESIUM	370mg
CALCIUM	670mg

PUMPKIN SEEDS

Helps lower cholesterol levels ◆ Have anticancer effects

Good source of omega-3 fats and zinc

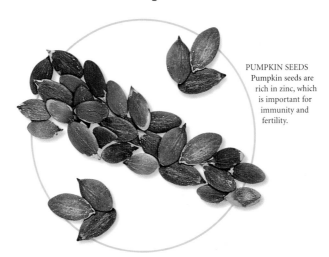

PUMPKIN SEEDS
Pumpkin seeds are
rich in zinc, which
is important for
immunity and
fertility.

MAXIMIZING THE BENEFITS

Phytosterols are found in seeds and nuts (and their oils), grains, and vegetables, and a plant food-based diet provides a good intake. Store seeds in a sealed container, preferably in the fridge. Avoid brown seeds, which may be rancid. Chew seeds well.

HOW MUCH TO EAT

One tablespoon weighs ½oz. Enjoy pumpkin seeds as a snack, in salads, rice dishes, and baking. Roasting or toasting (in a skillet) brings out their flavor.

KEY BENEFITS

Pumpkin seeds are a key source of phytosterol phytochemicals (plant sterols). Like all seeds, pumpkin seeds are also nutritional nuggets (seeds are especially nutrient-rich for germination).

● **CHOLESTEROL LEVELS**
Phytosterols have a structure similar to cholesterol, and compete for absorption from the intestine. As a result, less cholesterol is absorbed, and cholesterol levels are lowered.

● **CANCER**
Laboratory and animal studies indicate that phytosterols can inhibit cancer development in colon, breast, and prostate cells. They may also help prostate problems.

● **HEART HEALTH**
Pumpkin seeds are also a good source of omega-3 fats, phytoestrogens, vitamin E, magnesium, and folate – all heart-healthy nutrients.

PUMPKIN SEEDS: OTHER PHYTOCHEMICALS

PHENOLIC ACIDS	pp.56–57
CAROTENOIDS	pp.72–73
LIGNANS	pp.54–55

NUTRITIONAL VALUES
Quantities per 4oz.

CALORIES	569
FIBER	5.3g
POTASSIUM	820mg
ZINC	6.4mg
IRON	10mg

ARTICHOKE

Promotes beneficial gut bacteria ◆ Helps reduce the risk of bowel upsets ◆ Good source of iron

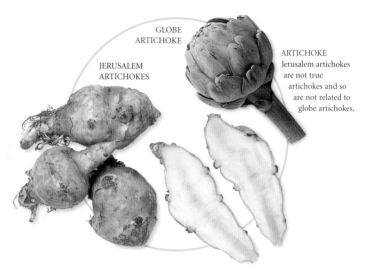

GLOBE
ARTICHOKE

JERUSALEM
ARTICHOKES

ARTICHOKE
Jerusalem artichokes
are not true
artichokes and so
are not related to
globe artichokes.

MAXIMIZING THE BENEFITS

Eating good sources of FOS daily (p.87) can help maintain a healthy balance of gut flora, which has other health benefits (p.21).

HOW MUCH TO EAT

An average serving of Jerusalem artichoke is about 4–5oz. Scrub well, boil, then peel. Serve with a little parsley and lemon juice or bechamel sauce, or purée or make into soup. Large globe artichokes need to be boiled for 30-40 minutes and should have the "choke" removed before being eaten.

KEY BENEFITS

Jerusalem artichokes contain a specific form of dietary fiber, fructo-oligosaccharides (FOS), which escapes digestion and is fermented by bacteria in the gut. FOS help beneficial lactobacilli bacteria to flourish in the gut. Globe artichokes are not rich in FOS, but extracts have cholesterol-lowering abilities (p.29).

● BOWEL UPSETS

Bowel upsets are often caused by the presence of harmful bacteria in the gut, which attach themselves to the gut wall and thrive. If FOS-rich foods stimulate the growth of

beneficial bacteria, they may block the attachment of harmful bacteria. FOS may also help reestablish beneficial bacteria after antibiotic treatment. These effects can be enhanced by eating a "probiotic" diet such as "live" yogurt. While FOS-rich foods can help, FOS supplemented foods will do more to actively change the gut flora (p.99).

ARTICHOKE: OTHER PHYTOCHEMICALS

FLAVONOIDS pp.34–35

NUTRITIONAL VALUES
Quantities per 4oz., raw

CALORIES	76
FIBER	1.6g
POTASSIUM	429mg
IRON	3.4mg

ASPARAGUS

May stimulate immunity ◆ May help lower cholesterol

Good source of folate and vitamin E

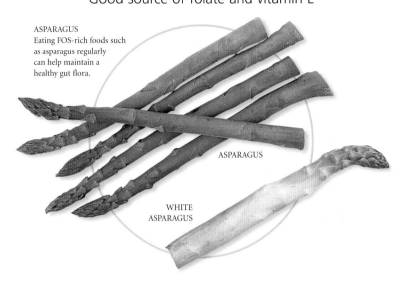

ASPARAGUS
Eating FOS-rich foods such as asparagus regularly can help maintain a healthy gut flora.

ASPARAGUS

WHITE ASPARAGUS

MAXIMIZING THE BENEFITS

Although FOS is not destroyed by cooking, conserve the excellent folate content of asparagus by steaming upright in a covered pan until just tender. Green asparagus contains more phyto-chemicals than white.

HOW MUCH TO EAT

An average serving of 5 asparagus spears weighs 5oz. Steam, char-grill, or roast fresh asparagus with olive oil and garlic. Canned asparagus still provides FOS, but tastewise is best used as part of a varied vegetable dish.

KEY BENEFITS

Asparagus is also a source of fructo-oligosaccharides (FOS), the special type of dietary fiber that promotes the growth of beneficial lactobacilli bacteria in the colon.

● IMMUNITY & CANCER

FOS has been shown to inhibit the growth of colon cancer cells in rats by stimulating their anti-cancer immune system. In another study, healthy humans given a daily ⅙oz supplement of FOS had increased numbers of beneficial bifidobacteria in their gut and significantly reduced levels of enzymes, which may promote cancer-causing agents.

● CHOLESTEROL LEVELS

FOS may help to regulate cholesterol levels. In one study, middle-aged men, who ate "live" lactobacilli yogurt with added FOS three times a day for three weeks lowered their cholesterol levels by 4.4 percent compared to those men who ate natural yogurt.

ASPARAGUS: OTHER PHYTOCHEMICALS

FLAVONOIDS	pp.34–35
CAROTENOIDS	pp.72–73
SAPONINS	p.103

NUTRITIONAL VALUES
Quantities per 4oz., cooked

CALORIES	13
FIBER	0.7g
FOLATE	74mcg
VITAMIN E	1.2mg

SEAWEED

Has anticancer effects ◆ Provides soluble fiber and

omega-3 fats ◆ Good source of iodine and selenium

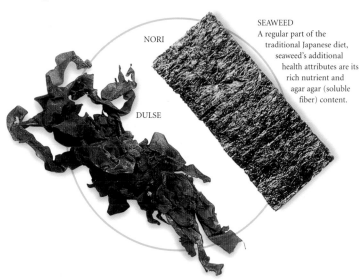

NORI

DULSE

SEAWEED
A regular part of the
traditional Japanese diet,
seaweed's additional
health attributes are its
rich nutrient and
agar agar (soluble
fiber) content.

MAXIMIZING THE BENEFITS

Iodine, needed for a healthy thyroid, and selenium may be lacking in the diet, especially vegetarian diets, so seaweed adds important nutrients.

HOW MUCH TO EAT

An average ⅜oz. portion of dried seaweed is very nutritious. Nori, the sweetest variety, is dried and then pressed into thin sheets. Buy ready toasted and use to wrap sushi (rice parcels filled with fish, pickle, avocado, or egg). Or crumble and garnish soups, salads, and stir fries.

KEY BENEFITS

Seaweed displays strong antioxidant activity. This is partly due to its fuco-xanthins; other phyto-chemicals responsible are still being identified.

● **BREAST CANCER**
Canadian scientists investigating low breast cancer rates among Japanese women propose that their protection may come from the iodine and selenium content in seaweed. In addition, animal studies indicate that iodine is transported from the blood into breast cells where it causes apoptosis (the triggering of cancer cells to essentially "commit suicide").

● **VITAMIN B12**
Seaweed contains vitamin B12, but most of it is in a form that cannot be used by the body. Vegans should get B12 from fortified foods, although they can benefit from the high levels of iodine in seaweed.

● **AGAR AGAR**
Agar agar, extracted from seaweed, is a vegetarian alternative to gelatin.

SEAWEED: OTHER PHYTOCHEMICALS

OTHER CAROTENOIDS pp.72–73

NUTRITIONAL VALUES
Quantities per 4oz.

CALORIES	136
FIBER	44.4g
IRON	19.6mg
IODINE	1470mcg

SHIITAKE MUSHROOM

Helps fight cancer ◆ Stimulates the
immune system ◆ May help lower cholesterol

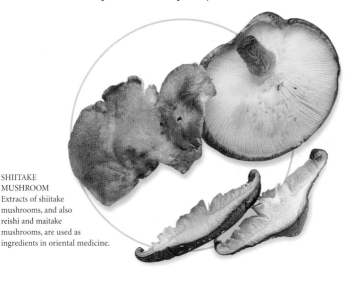

SHIITAKE MUSHROOM
Extracts of shiitake
mushrooms, and also
reishi and maitake
mushrooms, are used as
ingredients in oriental medicine.

MAXIMIZING THE BENEFITS

Only lentinan extracts
(as injections) have
been shown to exhibit
anticancer and anti-
viral benefits; while
there is no evidence
that eating shiitake
mushrooms will have
such effects, they do
contain good amounts
of B vitamins and
cholesterol-lowering
soluble fiber. Lentinan
is unaffected by heat.

HOW MUCH TO EAT

An average serving is
about 2oz. (a medium
mushroom weighs ½oz.).
Shiitake mushrooms
add rich "meaty"
flavor to soups, stir
fries, and pasta sauces.

KEY BENEFITS

Shiitake mushrooms con-
tain a distinct type of
polysaccharide, called
lentinan. Lentinan
extracts are reputed to
have many health benefits
and are famous in Japan
where they are used and
approved as anticancer
drugs, usually in conjunction with conventional
chemotherapy.

● CANCER

Research indicates that
lentinan stimulates the
immune system to release
natural killer cells and
macrophages that can
destroy cancerous cells
and help the body to
resist and fight off
different cancers.

● OTHER EFFECTS

Lentinan extracts can boost
immunity and increase
resistance to bacterial and
viral infections. Lentinan's
potential use in helping to
manage complications of
AIDS is currently being
researched. Dried shiitake
mushrooms and extracts
are used in traditional
oriental medicine to help
lower blood pressure
and cholesterol.

SHIITAKE MUSHROOM: OTHER PHYTOCHEMICALS

MONOTERPENES p.102

NUTRITIONAL VALUES
Quantities per 4oz.

CALORIES	42
FIBER	2g
FOLATE	25mcg

LEMON

Has anticancer effects ◆ Helps lower cholesterol levels
Good source of vitamin C

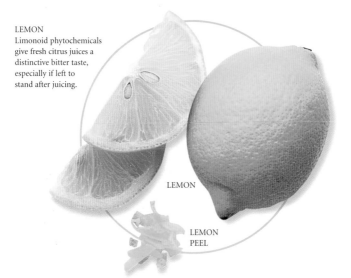

LEMON
Limonoid phytochemicals
give fresh citrus juices a
distinctive bitter taste,
especially if left to
stand after juicing.

LEMON

LEMON
PEEL

MAXIMIZING THE BENEFITS

Limonoids and limonene are found in the fruit, pith, peel, and juice (lemon rind and pith are the best sources), so make use of the whole lemon.

HOW MUCH TO EAT

Juice from a medium lemon makes about 2oz. Use in dressings, sauces, or as a drink. Scrub whole lemons and add the peel to fruit salads, rice salads, lemon sauces, and in baking. Aim to have a daily portion (p.19) of citrus fruit to benefit from this complete nutrient and phytochemical package.

KEY BENEFITS

Lemons and other citrus fruits are good sources of limonoid phytochemicals and a related phytochemical called limonene (a monoterpene). They both have recognized cancer-fighting effects.

● CANCER

Animal and laboratory studies reveal limonene's and limonoid's ability to block cancer development by stimulating "phase one and two" enzymes, which are part of the body's detoxification systems. Limonene may also inhibit cancer growth by triggering apoptosis (where cancer cells essentially commit suicide).

● CHOLESTEROL-LOWERING

Laboratory studies show that citrus limonoids have cholesterol-lowering properties, and researchers conclude that eating citrus fruits and products containing limonoids regularly may be a potentially important means to lowering cholesterol in humans.

LEMON: OTHER PHYTOCHEMICALS

| FLAVONOIDS pp.34–35 |
| PHENOLIC ACIDS pp.56–57 |

NUTRITIONAL VALUES
Quantities per 4oz., juice

CALORIES	7
FIBER	0.1g
POTASSIUM	130mg
VITAMIN C	36mg

GARBANZA BEANS

Help lower cholesterol levels ◆ Have anticancer effects

Good source of protein and folate

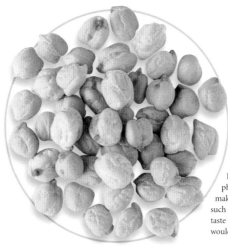

GARBANZA BEANS
High levels of the
phytochemical saponin
makes uncooked sources
such as garbanza beans
taste bitter, which deters
would-be predators.

MAXIMIZING THE BENEFITS

Dried garbanzas must be soaked overnight and boiled (in fresh water) until tender; or use canned ones. Eat garbanzas and other legumes regularly to benefit from their saponin, isoflavone, protein, fiber, iron, and folate content.

HOW MUCH TO EAT

One serving of cooked garbanzas is 4oz. Use in soups, salads, or casseroles, or in place of meat. Puréed garbanzas are the basis for the classic Middle Eastern dishes hummus and falafel.

KEY BENEFITS

Garbanzas – and other legumes such as soy beans and bean sprouts – are sources of a group of phytochemicals called saponins. Saponins can act as antioxidants, with a range of potential benefits.

● **CHOLESTEROL LOWERING**
In studies, saponin-rich alfalfa extracts have been shown to lower cholesterol levels. Saponins bind bile acids and cholesterol in the gut and reduce their absorption (bile acids are made from cholesterol, which is broken down to replace the lost bile acids, so cholesterol levels fall). Garbanzas also contain cholesterol-lowering soluble fiber and fructo-oligosaccharides.

● **CANCER**
Studies indicate that saponins have anticancer effects by blocking the development of cancer cells and stimulating the immune system.

GARBANZAS: OTHER PHYTOCHEMICALS

ISOFLAVONES pp.50–52	
FRUCTO-OLIGOSACCHARIDES pp.98–99	
PROTEASE INHIBITORS p.94	

NUTRITIONAL VALUES
Quantities per 4oz., boiled

CALORIES	121
FIBER	4.3g
PROTEIN	8.4g
FOLATE	54mcg

BANANA & PLANTAIN

Help maintain bowel health ◆ Good energy-boosting snack

Source of potassium and vitamin B6

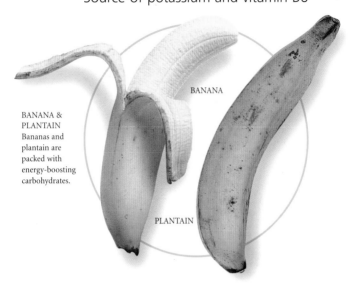

BANANA

BANANA &
PLANTAIN
Bananas and
plantain are
packed with
energy-boosting
carbohydrates.

PLANTAIN

MAXIMIZING THE BENEFITS

Ripe bananas are an excellent source of energy-boosting fruit sugars and make an ideal snack before, during, or after exercise. Fresh ripe bananas have the best nutrient content since plantain needs to be cooked in order to be palatable and digestible.

HOW MUCH TO EAT

One medium banana weighs 4oz. Use as a snack, on cereal, in sandwiches, and in desserts. Plantain, traditionally used in Caribbean cuisine, is generally cooked in nonsweet dishes.

KEY BENEFITS

Bananas and plantains are sources of two biogenic amines, serotonin and dopamine. Biogenic amines are also made in the body, and these forms of serotonin and dopamine can influence mood and appetite. Biogenic amines in food are inactivated by the enzyme monoamine oxidase in the gut lining, so are unlikely to have direct effects in the body. However, bananas are a good source of vitamin B6, which the body needs to make serotonin. Chocolate contains biogenic amines, too, but can boost moods because it tastes so good!

● BOWEL HEALTH

Plantains are rich in resistant starch (starch that is not digested), which can aid constipation. Diets rich in resistant starch are linked to lower incidence of bowel cancer. Ripe bananas are well-digested, and their fiber content provides bulk and aids regular bowel movement.

BANANA: OTHER PHYTOCHEMICALS

PHENOLIC ACIDS pp.56–57	
FRUCTO-OLIGOSACCHARIDES pp.98–99	

NUTRITIONAL VALUES
Quantities per 4oz., flesh

CALORIES	95
FIBER	1.1g
POTASSIUM	400mg
VITAMIN B6	0.3mg

COFFEE

Improves alertness ◆ Linked to reduced risk of Parkinson's disease ◆ Helps protect the body from free radicals

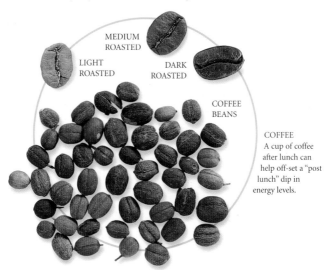

MEDIUM
ROASTED

LIGHT
ROASTED

DARK
ROASTED

COFFEE
BEANS

COFFEE
A cup of coffee after lunch can help off-set a "post lunch" dip in energy levels.

MAXIMIZING THE BENEFITS

The phenolic phyto-chemicals in coffee mean that moderate coffee drinking may bring benefits.

HOW MUCH TO EAT

An average cup of coffee is 4–6oz. Up to 2–3 cups of filtered coffee daily is considered moderate, with no firm evidence of harmful effects in healthy people. Those on medical advice and pregnant women should drink less. Remember that tea, cola, and chocolate also provide caffeine or related xanthine alkaloids.

KEY BENEFITS

Xanthine alkaloids are phytochemicals that have a mild stimulatory effect on the central nervous system. They include caffeine in coffee and tea, theophylline in tea, and theobromine in cocoa. Mild stimulation can be beneficial, but high intakes may affect sleep, trigger headaches, and anxiety-like symptoms. They also have a diuretic effect.

● ALERTNESS

Moderate coffee drinking can increase alertness and concentration, decrease fatigue, and improve performance for people working during the day or at night.

● PARKINSON'S DISEASE

A study that followed the diet and health of 8,000 Japanese-American men for 25 years found that men who drank five 5-oz cups of coffee a day were five times less likely to develop Parkinson disease compared to those who drank no coffee. Caffeine from non-coffee sources were also protective. More research is still needed in this area.

COFFEE BEAN: OTHER PHYTOCHEMICALS

FLAVONOIDS pp.34–35	
PHENOLIC ACIDS pp.56–57	

NUTRITIONAL VALUES
Quantities per 4oz., infusion

CALORIES	2
POTASSIUM	66mg

KIWIFRUIT

Has anticancer effects ◆ One of the world's most nutritious fruit ◆ Source of vitamin C and potassium

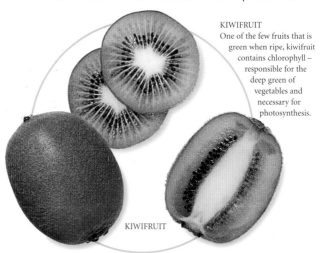

KIWIFRUIT
One of the few fruits that is green when ripe, kiwifruit contains chlorophyll – responsible for the deep green of vegetables and necessary for photosynthesis.

KIWIFRUIT

MAXIMIZING THE BENEFITS

Eat kiwifruit as soon as they are ripe (chlorophylls decrease with ripening), and slice just before eating to conserve the excellent vitamin C levels in the fruit.

HOW MUCH TO EAT

An average kiwifruit (flesh only) weighs 3oz. Eat kiwifruit like a boiled egg: cut in half and scoop the flesh out with a teaspoon. The tangy, sweet taste and vivid color of kiwifruit adds zest and nutrition to blended fruit juice, green salad, fruit salad, and dessert toppings.

KEY BENEFITS

Kiwifruit gets its green color from the phytochemical chlorophyll. It also contains actinidin, a plant enzyme *(p.107)*, and a wealth of nutrients and antioxidants. An American study ranked kiwifruit as the most nutritious of 27 popular fruit. Despite its name, kiwifruit originally came from China (and was called Chinese gooseberry), but New Zealand growers have popularized it worldwide.

● CANCER

When eaten, chlorophyll is converted to compounds (also found in green tea) that recent laboratory studies have shown to fight cancer by binding cancer-causing agents and inhibiting cell growth. Kiwifruit juice can also block the formation of nitrosamine (a potential cancer-causing agent) from nitrates in food *(p.109)*. This is probably due to its vitamin C and phytochemical content.

KIWI FRUIT: OTHER PHYTOCHEMICALS

FLAVONOIDS pp.34–35	
PHENOLIC ACIDS pp.56–57	
CAROTENOIDS pp.72–73	

NUTRITIONAL VALUES
Quantities per 4oz.

CALORIES	42
FIBER	1.6g
POTASSIUM	250mg
VITAMIN C	51mg

PINEAPPLE

May have anti-inflammatory effects ◆ Used as a meat tenderizer ◆ Useful source of potassium and vitamin C

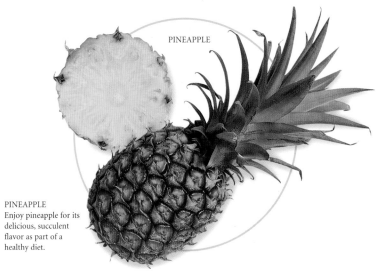

PINEAPPLE

PINEAPPLE
Enjoy pineapple for its delicious, succulent flavor as part of a healthy diet.

MAXIMIZING THE BENEFITS

Only small amounts of bromelain are found in the fresh fruit or juice, so eating pineapple on its own will not provide potentially helpful amounts. Cooking destroys bromelain, too. Enjoy pineapple for its succulent flavor and reasonable nutrient content.

HOW MUCH TO EAT

A thick slice weighs about 3oz. Choose fruit that smells sweet and pinappley. Cut off the peel, slice, and use as a snack, with cheese, or in rice salad, or fruit salad. It is delicious barbecued or flambéed.

KEY BENEFITS

Pineapple is famous for containing the plant enzyme bromelain. Bromelain breaks down proteins, and most is found in the stem rather than the fruit of the plant. Bromelain is used commercially as a meat tenderizer, and there has also been much interest in its potential medicinal uses as a supplement.

● **ANTI-INFLAMMATORY EFFECTS**
Like all enzymes, bromelain is made from protein. Any form of protein is usually digested, but when eaten with a meal, some bromelain may escape digestion and

be absorbed. A number of health claims have been made for bromelain supplements. These include anti-inflammatory effects that may alleviate joint pain and sinusitis, and reduce the risk of thrombosis. It is also suggested that they can aid digestion. More research is needed to verify such claims.

PINEAPPLE: OTHER PHYTOCHEMICALS

PHENOLIC ACIDS pp.56–57	
BIOGENIC AMINES p.104	

NUTRITIONAL VALUES
Quantities per 4oz.

CALORIES	41
FIBER	1.2g
POTASSIUM	160mg
VITAMIN C	12mg

GUIDE TO FOODS TO USE WITH CARE

Many different foods contain substances that could harm
our health. In most cases, problems only arise if excessive
amounts of an offending food are eaten, but in
some cases just small amounts can be toxic.

Food may contain certain substances
that could harm our health. Bad
reactions to foods may be caused by:
• A mycotoxin, which causes mold
and food spoilage,
• Contamination by harmful bacteria,
• Carcinogen formation such as
charred meat,
• Intolerance to a particular food
component, for example, gluten in
grains causing celiac disease,
• Certain phytochemicals.

SENSITIVITY AND INTOLERANCE

A small number of individuals are
sensitive to certain phytochemicals.
For example, sulfides in garlic can
lead to contact dermatitis or nausea;
capsaicin in chili peppers can
inflame the skin; caffeine in coffee
may trigger migraine; actinidin in
kiwifruit and bromelain in pineapple
can cause allergic reactions. About
two percent of the population have
some form of bad reaction to
foods, with dairy foods and wheat
being the biggest offenders. If you
find you are sensitive to something
such as kiwifruit, excluding it from
your diet is straightforward. If you

suspect more complicated food
intolerance, it is best to ask advice
from a qualified dietitian who will
make sure your diet is nutritionally
balanced in case you do need to
exclude foods.

Phytochemicals are present in
plants because they help them in
some way. As a natural defense, most
wild plants tend to be toxic or bad-
tasting to plant-eating animals. It
makes sense then that some phytochemicals may be harmful for us,
too. While some wild plants still
form an important part of traditional diets, they are rarely eaten in
developed countries. In fact, we only
eat a relatively small range of plant
species, which have been selected and
bred to make sure the ones we do eat
are low in natural or inherent toxins.

Plant breeding has allowed us to
enjoy essentially "safe," good-tasting,
and colorful plant foods. Low levels
of some compounds such as
tannins give a pleasing astringency
to foods, whereas more "wild" levels
would make foods inedible. One
downside of plant breeding is that
plants have lost much of their
natural ability to ward off pests, so

insecticides are needed to protect crops instead. In some cases, for example salicylates *(p.61)*, these natural plant healers may help our health, but reduced levels due to modern farming methods may be depriving us of this benefit.

NITRATES

Small amounts of nitrates are naturally found in plant foods but some, such as lettuce, spinach, and celery, contain fairly high levels as they accumulate nitrates from the soil (nitrates in soil are increased by nitrate-containing fertilizers).

Levels of nitrates in these vegetables are monitored by governments, and no health concerns have been identified. The potential concern over nitrates is that they can be converted to nitrites by bacteria in the gut, which in turn could combine with amines in the gut to form nitrosamines. Nitrates and nitrites are also used to preserve meats. Animal studies show that high levels of nitrosamines can be carcinogenic, but no link has firmly been established between nitrosamines and cancer in humans. The good news is that some nitrate in the diet may be beneficial, and a fruit and vegetable-rich diet is also rich in vitamin C and phytochemicals that block the formation of nitrosamines.

TOXIC PHYTOCHEMICALS

Phytochemicals either pass through the body undigested, or are absorbed, metabolized, and then able to react with the body's cells.

Some phytochemicals are toxic to cells, for example:

- Glycoalkaloids in green potatoes *(p.111)*,
- Cyanogenic glycosides in cassava or lima beans *(p.112)*,
- Pyrollizidine alkaloids in comfrey tea, which can damage liver cells and trigger cancer,
- Lathyrogens, associated with Indian lathyrus crops (a type of legume), which can damage brain cells and cause paralysis if eaten as a main part of the diet (primarily a problem in India),
- Hypoglycin in Jamaican ackee fruit, which can cause vomiting.

EATING IN EXCESS AND NEGATIVE EFFECTS

Aside from these extreme and easily avoided examples are the phytochemicals in foods that we commonly eat. In moderate amounts they are very beneficial, but in excessive amounts they may begin to have negative effects in the body. Examples include phyto-estrogens, glucosinolates, phytic acid, furanocoumarins, and xanthine alkaloids.

Eating just about anything in excess is not ideal, including specific nutrients such as vitamins, minerals, and fiber, especially if taken as self-prescribed high dose supplements. The same is probably true for phytochemical supplements *(see p.28)*. This all goes back to the importance of finding the right balance and variety of foods to provide us with a healthy, nutritious, plant-food based diet.

CAUTION

Phytoestrogens and salicylate phytochemicals have potentially beneficial effects, but some people need to take care.

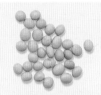

SOY BEANS

SOY BEANS are rich in isoflavone phyto-estrogens. The possibility that very high intakes of phytoestrogens might have side effects is currently being investigated, as are the safe upper limits for different age groups consuming phyto-estrogens in food.

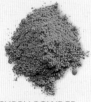

CURRY POWDER

CURRY POWDER is a rich source of salicylate, a phenolic acid that helps keep plants healthy by fighting off any infections. Despite salicylate's potentially beneficial effects, a small number of people may be sensitive to it, making curried food off limits for them.

PHYTOESTROGENS

In the 1940s sheep farmers in western Australia were hit by a breeding problem. Their ewes could not conceive, and the cause was found to be isoflavone-rich clover, which impaired their fertility. This raised the possibility that high intakes of phytoestrogens could have side effects in humans, too, for example, on thyroid function and fertility.

RESEARCH STUDIES

Until recently, there has been little research in this area; more information is needed. While essentially precautionary, any health effects on babies fed solely on soy-based formula milk before being weaned are being investigated. Meanwhile, the current advice is to give babies soy infant formula only on the advice of a health professional. It is almost impossible to eat enough phytoestrogen-rich foods to get close to the amounts eaten by sheep. Also, the amounts generally recommended for specific health benefits are considered "safe" (see also p.49). It is wise, however, to be wary about high-dose isoflavone supplements; women who have had breast cancer or who are at high risk should seek advice from their doctor.

SALICYLATES

Salicylate is a type of phenolic acid that plays an infection-fighting role in plants. Studies suggest it may help to reduce the risk of bowel cancer in humans and also exert anti-inflammatory benefits (aspirin is derived from salicylate). However, a small number of people may be intolerant to high intakes of salicylate, and it has been implicated in some cases of asthma, eczema, and nettle rash. Such people are often intolerant to aspirin (which contains a lot of salicylate compared to foods). Recent work in Britain has identified a number of people with "Sampters Triad," a condition where people have asthma, nasal polyps, and salicylate sensitivity. Minimizing salicylate in their diet helps control the asthma and nasal polyps. The general level of salicylate in the diet has been reduced by modern farming methods, but salicylate-rich foods include dried spices and herbs, menthol, berries, peppers, and oranges.

CAUTION

Some phytochemicals can reduce the absorption of minerals, and some are very toxic in large amounts.

OXALIC ACID

Very high intakes of oxalic acid (or oxalate) can be toxic, causing vomiting, diarrhea, and muscle cramps, but average dietary intakes of oxalic acid are not harmful. Plant foods such as rhubarb, spinach, and beet are rich in oxalic acid, while chocolate, cocoa, nuts, and tea are moderate sources. These foods are best limited in the diets of anyone suffering from oxalate-rich kidney stones. Oxalic acid may also bind and reduce the absorption of minerals, especially calcium, meaning that much of the calcium in spinach, for example, is not absorbed by the body.

PHYTIC ACID

Phytates – salts of phytic acid – are found in all plant foods as they are the plant's form of storing phosphates and other minerals. About 90 percent of phytates in our diet come from cereal-based foods, especially wholegrains. Legumes, seeds, and nuts are the other sources. While phytates have health benefits (see p.96), they can also bind with minerals such as iron, zinc, and calcium, reducing their absorption

into the body. Including vitamin C as part of a meal can help counteract the inhibition of iron absorption, and having a varied diet helps to optimize the absorption of minerals. However, try to limit raw bran, which is rich in phytic acid. It is better to get fiber and smaller amounts of phytic acid from a range of nutrient-rich wholegrains, seeds, and nuts eaten throughout the day.

GLYCOALKALOIDS

Very small amounts of glycoalkaloids are found in potatoes and other members of the nightshade family (tomatoes, eggplant, red and green peppers). These phytochemicals can be toxic in large amounts. Green and sprouted potatoes also have high levels of the glycoalkaloid solanine, and should be avoided. Store potatoes in a cool, dark place to prevent them from turning green. Green tomatoes also have relatively high levels of the glycoalkaloid solanine. Glycoalkaloid poisoning in the body causes vomiting and diarrhea, and if very severe, can prove fatal.

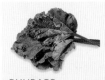

RHUBARB

RHUBARB is a rich source of oxalic acid. People with oxalate-rich kidney stones may need to restrict oxalic acid in their diet and should also drink plenty of fluids.

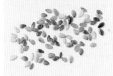

SESAME SEEDS

SESAME SEEDS are rich in phytic acid, which makes up about five percent of their weight. Eat with vitamin C-rich fruits and vegetables to aid iron absorption.

POTATOES

SPROUTING or green potatoes should not be eaten since they may contain harmful levels of glycoaloids. High intakes can become toxic in the body and cause severe vomiting and diarrhea.

CAUTION

Some phytochemicals reduce the amount of iodine absorbed from food; others need special preparation.

BRUSSELS SPROUTS

BRUSSELS SPROUTS and other cruciferous vegetables are classified as "goitrogens" – foods that, when eaten in large amounts, have the potential to cause goiter.

DRIED KIDNEY BEANS

EATING AS few as four or five raw kidney beans can trigger a reaction. Always soak raw, dried kidney beans in water for at least five hours, then boil for 15 minutes or more to destroy all the lectins.

CASSAVA

CONSUMING large amounts of cassava and lima beans raw can prove fatal. To avoid any toxic effects, cassava should be prepared correctly by being ground, washed, dried, and cooked before being eaten.

GLUCOSINOLATES

Glucosinolates are the phytochemicals found in cruciferous vegetables such as Brussels sprouts, cabbage, broccoli, and turnips. Very high intakes of these foods, especially raw cabbage, may cause a condition known as goiter (a swelling of the thyroid gland) in response to a reduced amount of iodine in the diet (glucosinolate derivatives can lower iodine absorption) and reduce the body's ability to make thyroid hormones.

IODINE INTAKE

Although goiter is rare in developed countries, anyone who eats cruciferous vegetables daily, especially vegans, should guarantee an adequate iodine intake. Iodine is found in dairy foods, seafood, seaweed, vegetables (depending on the iodine content of soil), and iodized salt. There is, however, no evidence that cruciferous vegetables cause harm as part of a varied diet – in fact, so far there is evidence only of their health benefits.

LECTINS

Raw kidney beans contain certain types of lectin phytochemicals that if consumed uncooked can cause a rapid onset of extreme nausea, vomiting, stomach pain, and diarrhea in individuals. Fortunately, recovery is usually rapid, and the symptoms generally pass after a few hours.

CYANOGENIC ALKALOIDS

Cassava and lima beans contain the phytochemicals known as cyanogenic alkaloids, which are broken down to form the toxin cyanide. Cyanide is broken down further into a compound called thiocyanate, which is also derived from glucosinolate-rich vegetables. Eating large amounts of these vegetables can result in goiter. Cyanide can also have direct toxic effects on the body.

PROPER PREPARATION

Cassava, a starchy, tuberous root vegetable from which tapioca is derived, is a staple food in a number of developing countries. Cassava must always be carefully prepared, then cooked well in order to destroy the cyanogenic alkaloid phytochemicals; lima beans must also be cooked thoroughly.

CAUTION

Some phytochemicals may interact with certain drugs. People on medication should inform their doctor of dietary changes.

TYRAMINE

Tyramine is a type of biogenic amine phytochemical *(see p.104).* Rich sources of tyramine include alcoholic drinks, broad bean pods, textured vegetable protein (TVP), yeast and meat extracts, cheese, game, and pickled herrings. Individuals who take an antidepressant drug called "monoamine-oxidase inhibitors" should avoid tyramine-rich foods as a reaction between the drug and tyramine will affect the nervous system. This can result in a rapid rise in blood pressure, flushing, palpitations, headaches, and nosebleeds. Some people report that tyramine-rich foods may also trigger migraines, but the reason is not clear.

FURANO-COUMARINS

Furanocoumarins are a type of coumarin *(p.71)* found in parsnips, celery, parsley, celeriac, carrots, citrus fruits, and legumes. They are known as phyto-alexin phytochemicals, meaning they are produced by plants in response to infection or stress, so helping to keep plants healthy. Coumarins appear to offer health benefits at moderate

intakes (the amounts found in a balanced diet), but tests with furano-coumarin extracts suggest that high intakes have the potential to make skin sensitive to PUVA light therapy (used to treat psoriasis), and possibly UVA rays from sunlight. However, these effects have not been found with typical or even high dietary intakes of food such as celery.

HYDRAZINE

Very small amounts of hydrazine phytochemicals are found in a wide range of mushrooms, including cultivated mushrooms. Questions have been raised about their safety since studies suggest they may act as carcinogens. Research into hydrazines and other phytochemicals in mushrooms continues, but in the meantime scientists consider current intake levels safe. Don't forget that, like all wild plant foods, varieties of wild mushrooms can frequently contain quite toxic phytochemicals (which in some cases could prove fatal if eaten). Make sure any wild mushrooms you eat are picked only by mushroom experts.

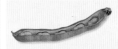

BROAD BEAN PODS

BROAD BEANS and their pods are one of a number of tyramine-rich foods that must be avoided by people taking the drug monoamine-oxidase inhibitors. A list of such foods is provided with this drug.

MUSHROOMS

HYDRAZINE levels, which are much lower in cultivated than wild mushrooms, are reduced further by storage and cooking. Current intakes are considered to be quite safe.

CELERY

FURANOCOUMARIN levels in foods such as celery and carrots decrease during cooking as they leach out into cooking water. They are not well-absorbed, and typical intakes do not pose any health risks.

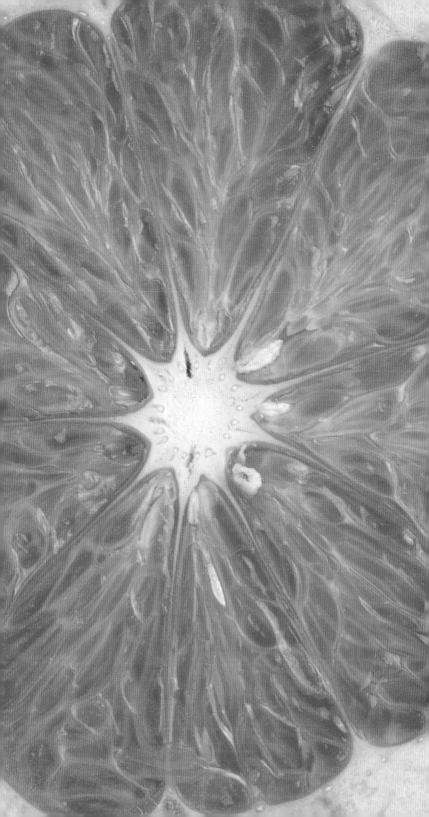

Part Three

Good food is vital for health. Our genetic

make-up influences health, but diet and lifestyle

shape it. Part Three highlights:

◆ Nutritional needs from birth to old age

◆ A guide to common conditions

◆ A glossary for scientific terms

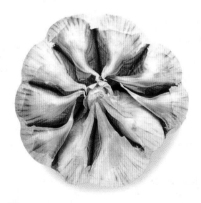

NUTRITIONAL NEEDS

Our nutrient needs and eating habits change dramatically through the first 20 years of life. One constant remains: nourishing food is needed to fuel growth and development and help every child achieve their unique potential.

BABIES

Breast milk is best for babies. It provides the optimal balance of nutrients needed for growth and development, and antibodies to build up immunity. Infant formula is available if parents choose not to, or are unable to, breastfeed.

Puréed fruit, vegetables, and rice cereals make ideal first foods; then variety and texture can be gradually increased. By six months of age they also need iron-rich foods in their diet.

KEY FOODS
◆ Breast milk or formula for first year.
◆ Start weaning from 4-6 months.
◆ Include iron and vitamin C-rich foods from 6 months *(p.23)*.
◆ Always use full-fat dairy foods and spreads when preparing baby food.
◆ Provide varied meals by one year of age.

HIGH-CALORIE DIET
Babies grow very quickly so they need plenty of calories packed in a small volume. While some fruit and vegetables are important, overdoing them may mean that babies don't get the calories they need. If they are gaining weight and growing as expected, they are doing well.

TODDLERS

Healthy toddlers are active. Three family-type meals plus suitable snacks will keep energy levels topped up. Full-fat cow's milk can be given as a main drink from 12 months; its calcium and vitamin D content are vital for growing bones and teeth. If they refuse milk, use calcium-rich alternatives. Children's vitamin drops are advisable unless you are confident that your toddler has a varied diet and gets outdoors often so vitamin D can be generated.

KEY FOODS
◆ Three meals plus snacks such as toast, fruit, cheese, vegetable sticks.
◆ At least two servings of calcium-rich foods such as yogurt, fortified soy milk or cow's milk, or cheese sauce.

PICKY EATERS
Toddlers can be picky eaters, but parents can allow them to follow their natural appetite and offer foods from each of the main food groups (see p.19) each day. Any sugary foods and drinks are best kept to mealtimes to avoid early tooth decay.

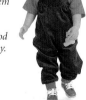

CHILDREN

School-age children are still growing, developing, and playing, and need good food for fuel. A plant food-rich diet *(p.19)* is now suitable as appetites are more robust, and its health-protecting powers are best if experienced over a lifetime. A child's early experience of food helps shape their eating habits in later life, so encourage them to enjoy a variety of tasty and nourishing foods. Relaxed family meals away from the television and other distractions helps develop the social side of food.

KEY FOODS

◆ A good breakfast that includes juice, cereal, milk, and toast.
◆ Nourishing packed lunches such as filled rolls or sandwiches, fruit, yogurt, a fruit bun or cereal bar, and a drink.
◆ Family meal whenever possible.

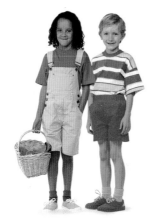

FUTURE HEALTH
Dietary surveys suggest that, in general, children eat too few vegetables, fruit, and dairy foods, and consume too many sweets, salty snacks, and sugary drinks. They have also become less active. This type of lifestyle could be sowing the seeds for potential health problems in the future.

TEENAGERS

Adolescence demands increased nutrition to cope with growth spurts and the onset of puberty. Around 95 percent of the maximum strength of the skeleton is established by late teens, and onset of menstruation means that girls' iron requirements almost double, and more protein, calcium, magnesium, and zinc are needed to build new tissue, muscle, and bone. Eating habits also change due to busy social lives, dieting, and experimentation with food trends.

KEY FOODS

◆ Iron-fortified breakfast cereal with milk and served with juice – eaten either as a speedy snack or as a nutritious breakfast.
◆ Other good snacks or quick meals include beans on toast, soup and a roll, nuts, dried fruit, fruit salad, cereal bars, peanut butter on wholemeal toast, pita bread and dips, fruit smoothies, yogurt or rice pudding, sandwiches, rolls, or wraps, and pasta or potato salad.

DIETS AND BODY IMAGE
Dietary surveys show that too many teenagers' diets, especially the diets of teenage girls, are low in the essential nutrients calcium, zinc, and magnesium, putting them at risk of energy-sapping anemia and osteoporosis in later life. Restricting nutritious food due to weight concerns is now known to be a common problem at this age.

NUTRITIONAL NEEDS

The adult years see the wonder of pregnancy, the hormonal changes of menopause, and the fragility of elderly years. At every stage food plays a vital role in optimizing health, vitality, and enjoyment as our bodies age naturally.

ADULTS

Although the adult body has stopped growing and developing, nutritional needs in these years remain high, and the beneficial effects of a plant food-based diet take on special importance. Maintaining a varied and phytochemical-rich diet, together with an active, tobacco-free lifestyle, reduces the risk of chronic disease, early aging, and day-to-day health upsets, and helps everyone look and feel their best.

KEY FOODS
- ◆ Five portions of fruit and vegetables daily.
- ◆ Three daily servings of wholegrain foods.
- ◆ Regular intakes of nuts, or legumes.
- ◆ Foods low in saturated fat and foods rich in omega-3 fats *(see Food Guide, pp.18–19, p.22)*.

AGING PROCESS
The longer we live, the more our bodies are exposed to free radicals, the effects of raised cholesterol, carcinogens in the environment, and illness.

PREGNANT WOMEN

Women who are planning a baby, or until the twelfth week of pregnancy, are advised to take a daily 400mcg supplement of folic acid and eat folic acid-rich foods to help reduce the risk of birth defects. Food rich in omega-3 fats *(p.22)* is important for a baby's developing brain, retina, and nervous system. Plant foods provide beneficial antioxidants.

KEY FOODS
- ◆ Folate and folic acid-rich foods: green leafy vegetables, legumes, orange juice, folic acid-fortified breads, cereals, yeast extracts.
- ◆ Omega-3 sources: oily fish, walnuts, rapeseed oil, pumpkin seeds, and wholegrains.

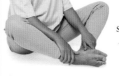

SPECIAL VALUE FOODS
Pregnancy doesn't mean having to "eat for two," but women do need to eat well before and after conceiving. Calories need rise only during the last three months of pregnancy, and increased nutritional needs can be met by a good-quality diet.

◆ Iron-rich foods: red meat, whole-grains, fortified cereals, greens, dried fruit, oily fish.

◆ Calcium-rich foods: milk, yogurt, cheese, calcium-fortified soy foods, and vitamin D via sunlight.

POSTMENOPAUSAL WOMEN

Women enter menopause when estrogen levels decline. Menopausal symptoms can be difficult and up-setting: cholesterol levels increase, bone strength declines, and body fat tends to gather around the waist. Almost one in four women will die of heart disease. A varied, plant food-rich diet can help to manage many of these potential problems.

KEY FOODS

◆ Phytoestrogen (and fiber)-rich foods such as soya foods, lentils, chick peas, other legumes, bean sprouts, linseeds, pumpkin seeds, and wholegrains.

◆ Calcium-rich foods: low-fat milk and dairy foods, fortified soy foods.

◆ Foods low in saturated fat and foods rich in omega-3 fats *(p.22)*.

◆ At least five portions of fruit and vegetables daily.

POSTMENOPAUSAL WOMEN
Phytoestrogen-rich foods may help the heart and menopausal symptoms. Adequate calcium and vitamin D levels, combined with weight-bearing activity, can help to minimize the loss of bone strength.

ELDERLY PEOPLE

As we age, calorie needs often decline, due to a drop in metabolism and less physical activity. However, some vitamin and mineral needs increase as the body uses them less efficiently. Natural antioxidant defenses decline too. A varied plant food-rich diet provides protective phytochemicals and should meet nutritional and fiber needs. But problems can start if interest in food wanes because of poor appetite, a limited budget, loneliness, illness, bereavement, or medication. A weekly check on weight helps flag any unhealthy weight loss when extra medical and nutritional help may be needed.

KEY FOODS

◆ Plant foods for antioxidants and zinc-rich foods (seafood, dairy foods, lean meat, wholegrains) - both for the immune system.

◆ Vitamin D - from oily fish, fortified foods, cheese, and eggs, or a daily supplement.

◆ Fiber-rich foods - wholegrains, linseeds, vegetables - plus at least 6 drinks daily.

◆ Small, frequent meals and nutritious snacks, and maybe a multivitamin and mineral supplement.

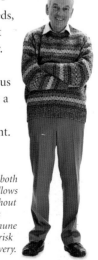

KEEPING HEALTHY
Staying active benefits both body and mind, and allows a good food intake without weight gain. This helps maintain a strong immune system, which reduces risk of illness and aids recovery.

QUICK
REFERENCE

Diet can help prevent or relieve a number of common ailments, and a healthy, balanced diet is the best starting point. Always seek individual medical and dietary advice to make sure you get tailor-made help for your health.

CONDITION	HELPFUL PLANT FOODS	TIPS/ADVICE
BOWEL HEALTH There are different types of bowel disorders that can be helped by diet. Regular meals, adequate fiber intake (some bodies are sensitive to too much), and stress management all help.	Fructo-oligosaccharide-rich foods and wholegrains. All fruit and vegetables, nuts, and seeds for different types of fibers and phytochemicals to help the bowel in different ways.	Drink at least 6-8 glasses of fluid daily. Eat live yogurt regularly. Limit seeds, skins, and bran if bowel is sensitive to fiber. Seek medical advice if your bowel habit changes noticeably.
CANCER Cancer is abnormal, unrestrained cell growth in an organ or tissues, often triggered by a carcinogen, which invades healthy tissues. Up to a third of cancers may be prevented by a healthy diet.	Have 5-9 portions of fruit and vegetables and 3 wholegrain foods daily. Many plant foods offer protection, especially wholegrains, cruciferous vegetables, nuts, garlic, citrus fruit, and legumes.	Eat red and processed meat in moderation. Keep to a healthy weight and moderate alcohol limits. Don't smoke; stay physically active. Don't eat charred meat. Limit smoked, pickled, and cured foods.
CATARACTS Cataracts are caused by changes to the fine proteins in the fibers in the lens of the eye. Oxidative stress is one possible cause.	Foods rich in carotenoids, especially lutein and zeaxanthin, eaten at least 4 to 5 times a week.	A regular intake of carotenoid-rich foods and vitamins C and E may also reduce the risk of age-related macular degeneration.

CONDITION	HELPFUL PLANT FOODS	TIPS/ADVICE
DIABETES Type 2 diabetes – the most common form – is a condition where there is too much glucose in the blood due to insufficient insulin. It affects people over 40, runs in families, and obesity increases the risk of developing it.	Carotenoid-rich foods – deep red, orange, and green fruit and vegetables for antioxidants. Foods rich in soluble fiber and with a low glycemic index – oats, beans, fruit, rye, lentils, pasta, and rye bread.	Eat at least 5 portions of fruit and vegetables daily and include wholegrains. Have at least one portion of oily fish weekly; cut saturated fat; eat regular meals; stay active; keep to a healthy weight.
GENERAL AGING Aging is not an ailment but a normal process that basically involves a reduction of the number of healthy cells in the body over time, which affects body functions.	All phytochemicals could play a role in delaying the physical effects of aging via the biological actions outlined in Part Two. A varied diet is vital.	Can a lifetime's diet rich in antioxidants delay aging and help people live longer, healthier lives? Some scientists think so, and the research continues.
HEART HEALTH Atherosclerosis causes coronary heart disease. Risk factors include: high cholesterol, smoking, high blood pressure, obesity, poor diet, lack of exercise, diabetes, and family history.	Foods high in soluble fiber (oats, rye, legumes, fruit,), nuts, garlic, food rich in flavonoids, folate (greens, wholegrains, legumes), phytosterols, fructo-oligosaccharides, tea, and red wine.	Choose unsaturated fats. Eat at least 5 portions of fruit and vegetables daily and include wholegrain bread and cereals. Eat oily fish 1-2 times per week. Be active for 30 minutes a day.
IMMUNITY The strength of the immune system to fight disease and cancer can be aided by a good supply of vitamins A, B6, C, E, zinc, iron, selenium, copper, and also phytochemical antioxidants.	Foods rich in flavonoids and other phenolic compounds. Foods rich in carotenoids. Garlic and onions. Plant foods also provide vitamins A (via carotenoids), C, E, and zinc.	Eat a balanced diet that includes at least 5 portions of fruit and vegetables daily, and wholegrains. Include food rich in omega-3 fats. Maintain a healthy weight and stay active.

CONDITION	HELPFUL PLANT FOODS	TIPS/ADVICE
LUNG FUNCTION Every time we breathe, large amounts of oxygen pass through the lungs, which over time may increase the risk of free radical damage to the cell membranes, inflammation, airway constriction, and wheezing.	Foods rich in flavonoid, phenolic, and carotenoid antioxidants (for vitamin C as well as phytochemicals). Wholegrains, vegetable oils, and nuts for selenium, and vitamin E (which form part of the antioxidant defense system).	Eat a balanced diet that includes at least 5 portions of fruit and vegetables daily, and wholegrains. Include foods rich in omega-3 fats. Limit salt and salty foods (excess salt may worsen existing asthma).
MENOPAUSE Most women in the West suffer menopausal symptoms to some extent – including hot flushes, dry skin, mood swings, fatigue – which are all influenced by hormonal changes. Risk of heart disease and osteoporosis is also increased due to these hormonal changes.	Foods rich in phytoestrogens – soya foods, linseeds, lentils, garbanza beans and other legumes, wholewheat, sprouts, and greens. Foods rich in soluble fiber. Plant food sources of calcium – greens, legumes, nuts, fortified soy foods.	Eat at least 5 portions of fruit and vegetables and include wholegrains daily. Limit saturated fat; choose foods rich in omega-3 fats. Include calcium-rich foods. Stay physically active and include weight-bearing exercise, which is best for keeping bones strong.
NERVOUS SYSTEM Exposure of the brain to long-term free radical attack to the brain is a strong candidate for increasing the risk of stroke and degenerative problems such as Alzheimer's and Parkinson's disease. The brain is more vulnerable to oxidative stress than other parts of the body.	A lifetime's intake of good sources of antioxidant nutrients and phytochemicals such as foods rich in flavonoids, other phenolic compounds, carotenoids, and garlic. See page 23 for guidance on which foods contain antioxidant vitamins and minerals.	Include at least 5 portions of fruit and vegetables daily and also include wholegrains. Include sources of omega-3 fats. For strokes, see Heart Health column. Recent research suggests a healthy diet low in saturated fat also reduces the risk of dementia.

CONDITION	HELPFUL PLANT FOODS	TIPS/ADVICE
OSTEOPOROSIS Affects 1 in 3 women and 1 in 12 men in their lifetime. Makes bones brittle and easy to break. Bones strengthen until the thirties, then gradually thin. Bone loss increases at menopause.	Foods rich in flavonoids and phytoestrogens. Calcium-rich plant foods – kale, bok choi, dried fruit, soy foods, legumes. Eat at least 5 portions of fruit and vegetables daily.	Make sure adequate calcium and vitamin D and balanced diet. Do regular weight-bearing exercise. Avoid being too thin. Moderate alcoholic intake.
RHEUMATOID ARTHRITIS Inflammation of joints, causing much pain and stiffness. Exact cause is not known, but may be an auto-immune disease. It affects people of all ages. Seek medical advice for treatment.	Foods that have phytochemicals with anti-inflammatory and anti-oxidant benefits may be helpful – e.g., phenolic and carotenoid-rich foods. Some people may have food intolerances.	Eat at least 5 portions of fruit and vegetables and include wholegrains daily. Limit saturated fat and choose virgin olive oil or rapeseed oil. Eat oily fish at least two times a week.
SKIN HEALTH Free radical damage to collagen (skin proteins) influences skin aging. Sunlight exposure and tobacco increase the skin's free radical exposure.	Carotenoid-rich foods – orange, red, and green fruit and vegetables, (also for vitamin C). Nuts, seeds, and wholegrains for selenium, zinc, and vitamin E.	At least 5 daily portions of a variety of fruit and vegetables as part of a balanced diet. Include foods rich in omega-3s. Drink at least 6 to 8 glasses of fluid daily.
WEIGHT CONTROL Weight is gained when we take in more calories from food and drink than we expend via our metabolism and levels of activity. Being obese (very overweight) increases the risk of heart disease, joint pain, infertility, and diabetes.	Most vegetables and fruit are tasty, filling, and low in calories. Snacking on fruit and eating decent quantities of vegetables can help manage weight. Plant foods rich in soluble fiber help regulate appetite, too.	There are three main aspects to regulating weight: a balanced diet, regular physical exercise, and healthy eating habits (i.e. feeling in control of your eating, especially comfort eating, being aware of the benefits of nutrition).

GLOSSARY

ALZHEIMER'S DISEASE: A progressive degenerative disease of the brain involving loss of memory and speech, and confusion.

ANTIOXIDANT: Antioxidants neutralize free radicals. Different types are needed to work in various body cells, and many work together. Some are produced by the body, such as glutathione peroxidase; others come from the diet (vitamins C and E, carotenoids, lipoic acid, flavonoids, and other phenolics).

ATHEROSCLEROSIS Thickening or furring up of the lining of artery walls, caused by cholesterol-rich deposits (atheroma). This leads to narrowing of the arteries, which may cause angina, and increases the risk of thrombosis. If a blood clot blocks the blood flow to the heart or brain it can trigger a heart attack or stroke. If "bad" LDL cholesterol is damaged by free radicals, it more readily thickens arterial walls. Antioxidants may protect against atherosclerosis by inhibiting LDL damage and inflammation of the arterial wall.

AUTO-IMMUNE DISEASE Disease caused by the body's immune system attacking its own tissues.

CARCINOGEN Any agent or substance that can produce cancer, e.g., certain industrial chemicals, cigarette smoke, sunlight exposure, alcohol, radiation, compounds in charred meat.

CHOLESTEROL A fatty substance made mostly by the liver and used to make cell membranes, hormones, and bile acids. Since fats don't dissolve in the blood, they must be carried by special proteins called lipoproteins: LDL (low density lipoprotein), and HDL (high density lipoprotein). "Bad" LDL cholesterol delivers cholesterol to the arteries; "good" HDL cholesterol carries cholesterol away from the arteries.

DNA (DEOXYRIBONUCLEIC ACID) An individual's genetic blueprint for their development and makeup.

DIURETIC Any drug or compound that causes a greater amount of fluid to be lost in the urine.

ENZYMES Catalysts that enable specific reactions to take place in the body.

ESSENTIAL FATTY ACIDS Types of polyunsaturated fatty acids that are essential to life, but can't be made in the body and must come from food. They are the omega-6 fatty acid, linoleic acid, and the omega-3 fatty acid, alpha-linolenic acid *(see p.22)*.

ESTROGENS Produced mainly by the ovaries in women, estrogens are needed for female sexual development and healthy reproduction. The adrenal glands produce small amounts of estrogen in both men and women.

FREE RADICALS Highly unstable molecules usually produced during chemical reactions in the body that involve oxygen, e.g., superoxide anion. They stabilize themselves by attacking other molecules, which can damage cells in the body.

IMMUNITY The body's ability to recognize and defend itself against foreign invaders such as bacteria, viruses, proteins, or damaged cells. Some phytochemicals help immunity by protecting immune system cells from the free radicals produced as part of their defensive reactions.

INFLAMMATION The body's response to damage caused by infection, injury, chemicals, temperature extremes, radiation, or free radicals. Some phytochemicals help control inflammation by influencing "cytokines" and eicosanoids *(p.22)*, and by neutralizing free radicals.

METABOLISM All the chemical reactions that occur in every cell in the body to sustain life and allow the body to function. These functions rely on nutrients and oxygen.

OXIDATIVE STRESS Excessive exposure to free radicals that can lead to damage in the body.

PARKINSON'S DISEASE A degenerative disorder of nerve cells in the brain that gradually leads to increased muscle tension and tremors, joint rigidity, and slow movements in the limbs.

PLATELETS & AGGREGATION Tiny blood cells in the body that play a role in blood clotting by aggregating (clumping together) in response to injury to a blood vessel wall, e.g., by damaged (oxidized) "bad" LDL cholesterol. Over time this contributes to atherosclerosis. If the injury is caused by ruptured atheroma it can trigger thrombosis.

PHOTOSYNTHESIS The process by which plants use their chlorophyll (green pigment in plants) to trap the sun's energy and make carbohydrates from carbon dioxide and water.

RISK FACTORS Factors linked to an increased likelihood of a disease, but not proven to directly or inevitably cause it.

SAFETY A scientific judgment that considers the risks to be acceptable.

THROMBOSIS The formation of a blood clot inside a blood vessel, which, if large enough, can block blood flow. High cholesterol levels (and atherosclerosis), inflammation, oxidative stress, smoking, diabetes, inactivity, and high blood pressure can all increase the risk of developing thrombosis.

TOXINS Poisons produced by bacteria, plants, or animals that cause harm by disrupting the function and/or the structure of cells in the body.

TRANS FAT Formed when unsaturated oils are "hardened" to make hydrogenated vegetable oils.

INDEX

REFERENCES & ACKNOWLEDGMENTS

Wayne R Bidlack et al. **Phytochemicals as bioactive agents**. Technomic Publishing Company, 2000; World Cancer Research Fund and American Institute for Cancer Research. **Food, Nutrition and the Prevention of Cancer: a global perspective**, 1997; Nutritional Enhancement of Plant-based Food in European Trade (NEODIET). Special Issue. **Journal of the Science of Food and Agriculture 2000**; 80: Issue 7; Oliver Gillie. **Food for Life: Preventing Cancer Through Healthy Diet**. Hodder and Stoughton, 1998.; JS Garrow and WPT James. **Human Nutrition and Dietetics**, Ninth Edition. Churchill Livingstone, 1993.; The National Academy of Sciences. **Dietary Reference Intakes for Vitamin C, Vitamin E, Selenium, Beta-Carotene and other Carotenoids.** The National Academy Press, 2000.; EN Whitney et al. **Understanding Normal and Clinical Nutrition.** Wadsworth Publishing Company, 1998; McCance & Widdowson. **The Composition of Foods**, Fifth Edition plus supplements. Royal Society of Chemistry and Ministry of Agriculture, Fisheries and Foods, 1995-1999; Ministry of Agriculture, Fisheries and Food. **Food Portion Sizes**. Second Edition. London: HMSO, 1994; John R Smythies. **Every Person's Guide to Antioxidants.** Free Association Books, 1998; Department of Health. **Nutritional Aspects of Cardiovascular Disease, Report on Health and Social Subjects Number 46,** London: HMSO, 1994; Department of Health. **Nutritional Aspects of the Development of Cancer, Report on Health and Social Subjects Number 48,** London: HMSO, 1998; Ministry of Agriculture, Fisheries and Food. **Inherent Natural Toxicants in Food: Food Surveillance Paper 51,** London: HMSO, 1996; C Rice-Evans. **Wake up to Flavonoids.** International Congress and Symposium Series 226. The Royal Society of Medicine Press Limited, 1999; Lampe JW. **Health effects of vegetables and fruit: assessing mechanisms of action in human experimental studies.** American Journal of Clinical Nutrition 1999; 70(suppl): 475-90S; Cantuti-Castelvetri I et al. **Neurobehavioral aspects of antioxidants in aging.** International Journal of Developmental Neuroscience 2000 ; 18: 367-381; M. Rhodes and KR Price. **Phytochemicals: Classification and Occurrence.** In: The Encyclopaedia of Nutrition 1539-1549, Academic Press, 1998; Rowland I. **Optimal nutrition: fibre and phyto-chemicals.** Proceedings of the Nutrition Society 1999; 58: 415-419; Block G et al. **Fruit, vegetables and cancer prevention: A review of the epidemiological evidence.** Nutrition and Cancer 1992; 18: 1-29; Steinmetz KA et al. **Vegetables, fruit and cancer prevention: A review.** Journal of the American Dietetic Association 1996; 96: 1027-1039; Hertog MGL et al. **Dietary antioxidant flavonoids and risk of coronary heart disease: the Zutphen Elderly Study**. The Lancet 1993; 342: 1007-1001; Bravo L. Polyphenols: **Chemistry, Dietary Sources, Metabolism, and Nutritional Significance**. Nutrition Reviews 1998; 56 (11), 317-333; Craig WJ. **Health-promoting properties of common herbs.** American Journal of Clinical Nutrition 1999; 70(suppl): 491-9S; Setchell KDR and Cassidy A. **Dietary Isoflavones: Biological Effects and Relevance to Human Health.** Journal of Nutrition 1999; 129: 758S-767S; World Health Organisation. **Diet, Nutrition and the Prevention of Chronic Diseases**. Report of a WHO Study Group. WHO: Geneva, 1990.

AUTHOR'S ACKNOWLEDGEMENTS: I would like to thank Liza Buckley, University of Leeds for her help with research, as well as the many scientists who provided information, especially Professor George Truscott, Keele University, Professor Alan Crozier, University of Glasgow, Dr Andrea Day and Dr Gary Williamson, Institute of Food Research, Norwich, Professor Mike Clifford, University of Surrey and NEODIET (Nutritional Enhancement of Plant-based Food in European Trade). Thanks, too, of course to Susannah Steel and Alison Lotinga for their good humour and great skills. Finally, thanks to Steve for his love and encouragement.

DK WOULD LIKE TO THANK: Peter Anderson, Ian Bagwell, Paul Bricknell, Geoff Brightling, Martin Cameron, Andy Crawford, Geoff Dann, Philip Dowell, Neil Fletcher, Peter Gardner, Steve Gorton, Dave King, Ranald Mckechnie, David Murray, Martin Norris, Stephen Oliver, Daniel Pangbourne, Roger Phillips, Tim Ridley, Jules Selmes/Debi Treloar, Clive Streeter/Patrick McLeary, Paul Venning, Colin Walton, Matthew Ward, Andrew Whittuck, Philip Wilkins, Michel Zabé for photography. Denise O'Brien, Melanie Simmonds, Marcus Scott at the DK Picture Library. Hilary Bird for the index. Maggi McCormick for American adaptation.